OXYGEN
TO THE
RESCUE

OXYGEN TO THE RESCUE

*Oxygen Therapies, and How
They Help Overcome Disease
and Restore Overall Health*

PAVEL I. YUTSIS, M.D.

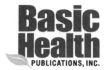

Basic
Health
PUBLICATIONS, INC.

The information contained in this book is based upon the research and personal and professional experiences of the author. It is not intended as a substitute for consulting with your physician or other healthcare provider. Any attempt to diagnose and treat an illness should be done under the direction of a healthcare professional.

The publisher does not advocate the use of any particular healthcare protocol but believes the information in this book should be available to the public. The publisher and author are not responsible for any adverse effects or consequences resulting from the use of the suggestions, preparations, or procedures discussed in this book. Should the reader have any questions concerning the appropriateness of any procedures or preparation mentioned, the author and the publisher strongly suggest consulting a professional healthcare advisor.

Basic Health Publications, Inc.
28812 Top of the World Drive
Laguna Beach, CA 92651
949-715-7327 • www.basichealthpub.com

Library of Congress Cataloging-in-Publication Data

Yutsis, Pavel.
  Oxygen to the rescue : oxygen therapies, and how they help overcome disease and restore overall health / Pavel Yutsis.
    p. ; cm.
Includes bibliographical references and index.
  ISBN-13: 978-1-59120-007-9
  ISBN-10: 1-59120-007-5
  1. Oxygen therapy.
  [DNLM: 1. Hyperbaric Oxygenation. 2. Complementary Therapies.
3. Hydrogen Peroxide—therapeutic use. 4. Ozone—therapeutic use.
5. Ultraviolet Therapy. WB 342 Y95o 2002] I. Title.

RM666.08Y88   2003
615.8'36—dc21

                                            2003000129

Editor: Roberta W. Waddell
Typesetter/Book design: Gary A. Rosenberg
Cover design: Mike Stromberg

Printed in the United States of America

10   9   8   7   6   5   4   3   2

Contents

This book is dedicated to my father-in-law,
David Grinman, in loving memory.
Our family will ever be grateful not only that
hyperbaric treatments extended his life for three years,
but also that each additional day he lived
was enhanced by oxygen and spent in an
ever-improving state of health.

I would also like to dedicate *Oxygen to the Rescue*
to former patients who have been returned to health,
and to all those who have yet to discover
the promise of oxidative therapies.

Acknowledgments

First and foremost, I would like to thank medical writer/editor Dee Ito for helping me shape new and often complicated information clearly and simply in a personal voice that is free from unnecessarily technical jargon. She understands very clearly that complementary approaches to medicine must first be understood if there is to be any possibility for broader acceptance. And toward that goal, I must also thank Roberta Waddell as project editor who not only shared Dee's insistence on clarity, but also used her insight and experience to bring in-depth attention to every detail of the manuscript. I believe our unique collaboration will contribute greatly to increasing public awareness of these very important oxidative therapies. My thanks to my publisher, Norman Goldfind, for his invaluable contribution to the overall concept of the book and for enthusiastically including it in the high-quality list of Basic Health Publications. Thanks also to Lee Clifford, MS, for her input in the beginning stages of research; and to Professor Joseph Dimant, my grateful appreciation for allowing me generous access to him and his knowledge of the science of neurology. To my lovely wife, Lilia, and my wonderful children, Max and Francine, thank you for your continuing love and support.

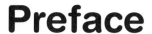

Preface

PRACTICING HEALING AS AN INTEGRATIVE MEDICAL DOCTOR

This is a book I have been wanting to write for a long time. The importance of pure oxygen as a treatment has been central to my medical practice from the very beginning, but it is just one part of what I do as an integrative complementary physician. Before exploring with you the value of the different oxygen therapies and what they can do, I'd like to explain some things about the way I practice medicine and also give you some background on the direction I've chosen. I am certainly not alone in this relatively new field of medicine that combines the use of conventional medical treatments—pharmaceuticals or surgery, for example, with alternative approaches, such as acupuncture, chelation, herbs and supplements, and oxygen therapies. There are many of us, and our numbers grow with each new medical school class. As with any new direction, however, these ideas and concepts need to become even more visible so the public will understand that conventional medicine is not the only choice for everyday medical care. We, in fact, believe it is best used *only* for acute emergencies.

In Russia, where I began my journey as a doctor, there were few distinctions between conventional and what we in the United States call alternative or integrative/complementary medicine. Medicine was medicine. Whatever approach worked to help a patient feel better, any treatment that would return an ill person to health was considered appropriate. And that made sense to me then, as it does now. In Russia's healthcare system at the time, it was a matter of necessity to use less expensive, more easily accessible treatments whenever possible. Those constraints forced Russian physicians to explore creative solutions for healing, and made it necessary to learn more about individual patients.

We, of course, discovered that most illness was a combination of problems, and that each needed to be considered if we were to return a patient to whole-body health. Examining natural and home remedies for possible application was not considered unscientific; hands-on bodywork was not out of the question; acupuncture was inexpensive and effective; and healthier diets, as well as vitamins and supplements, helped maintain strength while the body healed. We used all approaches, individually and together. The inability to regularly prescribe expensive technological solutions gave us new respect for simple solutions that were very often effective.

In the United States, where medicine was once rooted in natural approaches, the focus of medical achievement in the twentieth century has been on technology, and through the years, this direction has fostered the belief that the best medicine had to be expensive and technological. As physicians and patients, we have come to believe that *only* these approaches and treatments could keep people healthy, which has *not* turned out to be the case, even though we have all benefited greatly from access to new drugs and new surgical techniques. The new diagnostic equipment—CAT scans (computerized axial tomography), MRIs (magnetic resonance imaging), and mammography, among others—is a godsend for detecting disease before there are serious developments. However, there are many everyday chronic illnesses that assail people for long periods of time, which doctors—using conventional approaches—fail to diagnose and fail to cure. These are the illnesses that cost people personal stress and the possibility of productive lives. For society, they mean lost work time and an unnecessary financial burden. Chronic fatigue immune dysfunction syndrome (CFIDS), cytomegalovirus (CMV) and other viruses, allergies, atherosclerosis, cancer, metabolic diseases, and others are conditions that conventional physicians are not always able to successfully treat with drugs or surgery. And they are all serious risks to health that demand the time, creativity, and personal attention of physicians if they are to be diagnosed accurately and treated successfully. My years as a doctor have taught me that medicine is not only a science, but also an art. And as with all arts, it is one that it is impossible to practice without creativity and an open mind. It is also impossible to treat patients successfully without getting at the source of the problem, which requires astute detective work. And I can tell you that conducting an exploratory diagnostic process with a patient takes time, far more than the ten minutes per patient that most physicians can allow in their schedules.

Determining what a person does for a living, how he or she eats, what medications are used, what the psychological and emotional states are, if there is any possibility of allergies or heavy metal toxicity, all are important factors in helping me learn the root cause of why a patient is not feeling healthy. The process demands interest, curiosity, time, trial and error, and search and discovery. As a complementary physician, I approach each patient as a challenge. The easy cases do not come our way too often, and the solutions applied in conventional medicine, drugs, and/or surgery are almost always insufficient, as anyone with a chronic problem will tell you.

THE RETURN TO THE WHOLE-BODY APPROACH TO MEDICINE

In the early 1900s, there were American physicians who believed in naturopathic approaches to medicine, and they practiced alongside those who believed in surgery and drugs as a more efficient direction for medicine. But this easy relationship was soon ended by the movement toward specialization, technology, and prescription drugs that we think of as contemporary medicine today. As this movement got a foothold and gained momentum, the naturopathic movement disappeared, and the practitioners who used homeopathy, herbs, vitamins, nutrition, exercise, and hands-on bodywork were deprived of a professional community. Little did they know that, although it had been seriously marginalized in America, the approach they believed in was shared by others in Europe, the East, and my own native Russia.

It would take most of a century devoted to developing new technologies in the treatment of disease before naturopathic professionals and doctors had enough confidence and acceptance to once again make our strong case to people now deeply dissatisfied with the medical status quo. It would take rising healthcare costs, a nursing shortage, overworked doctors, and a hospital system unable to keep up with the demand for expensive technology-based treatment to weaken our belief in the established system. Ordinary people began to seek answers outside conventional medicine. In the waning years of the twentieth century, it was noted that 42 percent of all Americans were using some form of alternative medicine, enough for the United States to establish The National Center for

Complementary and Alternative Medicine. In 2001, *The New York Times* announced that "Congress has voted to give almost $90 million for studying the usefulness of such popular nontraditional remedies as acupuncture, food supplements, homeopathy and body manipulation."

Those of us who already knew how effective these treatments were—most of us had been prescribing them for at least the past two decades—used this renewed interest as an opportunity to step up our exploration of foods that have healing potential, find funding for more definitive research on the use of oxygen and chelation therapies, and discover more about the use of vitamins and herbs. We began to reexamine the medical approaches of Eastern cultures and discovered that they, like us, believed strongly that whole-body health was dependent on the mind/body connection. It further strengthened our conviction that we were on the right path.

The support for our convictions has given physicians like myself the opportunity to commit fully to complementary, or integrative, medicine. Our medical degrees give us the option to prescribe drugs and surgery, but we tend to recommend approaches and treatments, such as acupuncture, chiropractic, massage, nutrition, osteopathy, and oxygen therapies, that enhance the whole body first, all far less invasive, all producing far fewer side effects. Chronic degenerative conditions tend to develop because one or all of three physical events take place in the body: 1) The liver shows a diminished ability to detoxify. 2) Tissues and organs show inflammatory changes. 3) There is an increase in free-radical activity. Oxygen therapies, in many cases, rectify these conditions. And that brings me to the subject of this book.

Oxygen to the Rescue is organized into four parts, and the back of the book contains references, footnotes, and two appendices listing bio-oxidative organizations and therapeutic uses for the various oxygen therapies. The first three parts detail the four major oxygen therapies, and the last part explains how these therapies work together. They are as follows:

- *Hyperbaric Oxygen Therapy (HBOT)*. This therapy administers pure oxygen to patients at several times normal atmospheric pressure. Delivering oxygen to the cellular level has a positive effect on the whole body. HBOT is considered a preferred medical treatment for a number of conditions and diseases outlined in this book. But its less well-known use in the treatment of arthritis, cerebral palsy, HIV/AIDS, stroke, and other troubling illnesses of our time also holds great promise.

- *Hydrogen Peroxide and Ozone Therapies.* These therapies are closely allied. As oxygenators and oxidizers, they react easily with other substances and can destroy bacteria, viruses, and even some types of tumors. Hydrogen peroxide, administered intravenously, can be used to treat a broad range of diseases, among them acute and chronic infections, candidiasis, heart disease, rheumatoid arthritis, and stroke. Ozone therapy treats similar conditions.

- *Photoluminescence, or Ultraviolet Irradiation of Blood (UVIB).* This is not technically an oxygen therapy, but by exposing blood to ultraviolet rays, it greatly increases the capacity of blood to absorb and utilize oxygen to stimulate the immune system and destroy microorganisms. It is often used in combination with other oxygen therapies for maximum healing power.

- *How HBOT, Hydrogen Peroxide, and UVIB Work Together.* The last part discusses how using different oxygen therapies together can deliver a maximum amount of oxygen to all of the body's systems, and how these therapies work symbiotically to balance the body. By strategically applying oxygen's ability to enhance cells and heal diseased tissue, the entire body can be returned to full health.

The practice of healing, which is the appropriate definition for the work we do as doctors, relies on our diagnostic skills and our ability to choose treatments for our patients from the full range of existing modalities, both in the conventional and integrative complementary traditions. In many instances, a treatment program for an individual patient includes oxygen, and inevitably, oxygen comes to the rescue.

Introduction

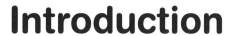

THE TRUTH ABOUT
OXYGEN THERAPIES

Starting out in medicine, I took oxygen therapies for granted. They were standard medical practice, as you might imagine, in a country where drugs and technological approaches to treatment were very expensive. But America presented me with a very different medical reality as I quickly realized that oxygen did not factor into medical treatment here. Most of my colleagues had little interest in the fact that many of my Russian patients had been routinely and successfully treated for the same chronic conditions and diseases that continued to plague their own patients. It's unfair to say that American doctors don't know anything about oxygen therapies. Most doctors are aware of hyperbaric oxygen therapy (HBOT), even if they seldom prescribe this treatment, because oxygen applied to the body under pressure is approved for use in limited situations such as carbon monoxide poisoning, poorly healed wounds, gas embolism, and decompression illness. Very few physicians, however, are aware that oxygen therapies have far more advanced medical applications that are commonly used in many countries outside the United States. In Russia, Europe, China, Japan, and Cuba, among others, oxygen therapies treat a broad range of conditions, such as arthritis, cancer, cerebral palsy, HIV, Lyme disease, optic neuritis, stroke, and even multiple sclerosis.

Experimenting with oxygen as a therapeutic treatment has been ongoing for more than 300 years, and curious researchers and committed physicians continue to be intrigued and excited by its potential. They wonder why applying increased oxygen to diseased cells in the human body revitalizes or changes the cell structure. Could this gas, a natural element, be used to treat disease with fewer side effects? Might supplemental oxy-

1

gen in the body actually repair cells or positively change their structure? How then to get more of it into the body? Are there ways to transport oxygen through the body more efficiently by using the body's own resources, or with the aid of herbs, vitamins, or other natural substances?

Coming some eighty years after the disaffection with the natural health movement began, the renewed interest in simple oxygen therapies as medical treatment is understandable. The accomplishments in medical science and technology that have produced breakthrough cures and diagnostic tools, that have improved the lives of millions of people, and that have given physicians the information they needed to do their work, are still not enough. Many of us are questioning why, in a time when complicated organ transplants are common, limbs get replaced with ease, and genetic engineering is a reality, human beings still have to experience chronic conditions and seemingly incurable diseases. It appears that technology does not have all the answers.

OXYGEN AND HOW IT WORKS IN OUR BODIES

The term *Oxygen Therapies* refers to all treatments that use oxygen to enhance the body's capacity to heal itself, as well as those that kill various bacteria, viruses, and other microorganisms that produce disease. When a therapy *adds* oxygen to blood or tissue, the clinical term is *oxygenation.* Hyperbaric oxygen therapy, referred to earlier, is an example of a therapy that uses oxygenation. The gas is placed under pressure, then forced into the body to increase the amount of oxygen reaching the cellular level.

Oxygen, the most abundant element in the atmosphere, is life, and without it, life would cease to exist. Yet, as we breathe it in and breathe it out, we have the luxury of taking it quite for granted because it is colorless, odorless, and tasteless, so we're seldom confronted with its vital importance to our physical and mental well-being. The air we breathe gives us the oxygen we need to live. The most important result of breathing for the body's continued functioning is a process called *oxidation*— when one atom or molecule loses electrons. The process whereby an atom or molecule accepts electrons is called *reduction.*

Oxidation occurs when oxygen combines with another substance, changing the chemical makeup of both. The easiest way to understand oxidation is the example of a log in a fireplace. By lighting it, we cause the wood to be oxidized, creating energy.

When we take in oxygen, our hearts, lungs, and circulatory systems carry it through our bodies, giving us the energy to function at an active level. Our lungs separate out the carbon dioxide (CO_2) from our blood, and it is expelled into the air. Preserving the environment becomes even more important when we realize that trees and plants are programmed to take in the carbon dioxide we eliminate from our bodies and turn it into the oxygen we use to breathe. The more trees, the more growing things around us, the more oxygen that is produced, so the health of our bodies depends on preserving as much of the natural environment as possible.

Under certain circumstances, however, life-sustaining oxygen can actually threaten life. Take, for example, cholesterol, a very important chemical compound in our bodies. Alone, *it causes no harm to our bodies*. In its natural state, it is an antioxidant. Antioxidants are chemical substances in vitamins, minerals, enzymes, and other elements that protect the cells and tissues of our bodies from the harmful influences of free radicals. Unlike stable molecules, free-radical molecules do not have paired electrons. In an effort to become stable, free radicals will steal an electron from a stable molecule, causing a chain reaction. One free-radical molecule can cause chemical changes in other molecules. Cholesterol *is* harmful, however, when it becomes oxidized, that is, when it is combined excessively with oxygen, which radically breaks down the molecular structure.

In his book *Oxygen and Aging*, Majid Ali says that "blaming coronary heart disease on healthy cholesterol is like blaming pure water for illness. Rancid cholesterol, like polluted water, can cause disease, so the focus must be on rancidity of cholesterol rather than on its blood level." Natural, non-rancid cholesterol is an antioxidant and, rather than causing harm to the body, a normal amount of it helps to protect the body by keeping it from producing an excess amount of free radicals.

The concern of the conventional medical community is that oxygen therapies, such as ozone and hydrogen peroxide, will cause cell damage, even mutations, because of the free radicals. Free-radical molecules are connected to the development of allergies, arthritis, cancer, diabetes, and other degenerative diseases, and contribute as well to immune deficiencies and the aging process. The healing objective in complementary medicine is to maintain the balance of molecules in the body in order to repair it and/or prevent disease. The positive side of free radicals is that they bring energy to the cells and kill bacteria, viruses, and fungi. We have to be concerned *only* when there is an excess number of free radicals, but in most healthy people, the body regulates the production of free radicals to prevent any excess. And in complementary medicine, where prevention of illness is at the core of our philosophy, we use various treatments, medications, and supplements in a continuing effort to maintain balance and help keep people healthy, and that includes keeping free radicals in check.

In my practice, I use oxygen therapies as my workhorses. Sufficient oxygen is indispensable to a healthy life. But a body fighting illness can use extra oxygen as a weapon to destroy viruses and bacteria, and to work at the cellular level in chronic conditions. I have seen cases of oxygen use bordering on the miraculous, where diseases and conditions have been reversed, and others where patients have been cured. Oxygen has the potential for giving new life to the cells in our bodies, and the exciting implications of that affects everyone, healthy people as well as those who are ill. Most of us have been in situations where access to fresh air is limited— long plane rides, closed concert halls packed with people, stuffy, airless rooms. Our bodies become tired, our energy is depleted, and sometimes we simply look and feel sick. Limited oxygen and an overexposure to carbon dioxide affects our physical well-being. However, healthy human beings return to normal as soon as we breathe in fresh air again. Our dependence on oxygen cannot be overemphasized. It is simple. Without oxygen, we cannot live. Inside a body deprived of adequate oxygen, the health of the entire body is affected at the cellular level (microorganisms are always on the lookout for low-oxygen environments where they can grow and develop into an illness). The first line of treatment in many emergencies is, in fact, the administration of oxygen through the nose, or by mask or ventilator.

Oxygen is 21 percent of the air we breathe and by learning to use this accessible, inexpensive element in healing, we can effectively treat a broad range of diseases and physical problems. The fact that it can be done with fewer (if any) side effects than most conventional treatments makes it a very attractive medical option.

The scientific link between low-oxygen environments and illness has long been known by researchers and physicians around the world. Many people have developed studies and treatment plans using oxygen to treat disease and the many chronic conditions that are so prevalent today. Oxygen is successfully used in the United States daily, but most physicians confine its usage to a narrow area, which we will discuss later.

Finding a cure for cancer has consumed us for most of the twentieth century and will continue to do so well into the twenty-first century. We have tried many directions in our search. And though we have certainly extended the life span of cancer patients, many of the conventional treatments have produced dangerous side effects. Oxygen therapy is not one of these. It is not toxic and has few, if any, side effects. Delivering oxygen to the cellular level has, in many cases, stabilized the progress of a disease while awaiting a true cure.

Cancer specialists, in particular, know that cancer cells grow in low-oxygen environments. These anaerobic microorganisms can be destroyed by the application of pure oxygen. Men and women with HIV/AIDS have been working with researchers in hopes that using oxygen treatments will help increase their T-cell counts or, at the very least, maintain their counts at an acceptable level. In North Carolina, John C. Pittman, M.D., has worked with HIV and AIDS patients, and his data shows that the hydrogen peroxide and ozone therapies he uses have helped a number of patients become HIV-negative.[1]

The advancements in medical science in the United States rank among the most innovative in the world. We enjoy the benefits of high-end technology and the newest drugs as soon as they become available. It's understandable, therefore, why we as patients and physicians are slower than the rest of the world to accept any treatment *not* developed or used here. Other nations, with fewer affordable options for the majority of its citizens, have been very bold in using HBOT as a primary treatment for a whole range of serious diseases. And in the process, they have compiled research that is beginning to interest more and more people in the United States, thereby increasing the demand for access to this treatment. Oxygen itself is inexpensive, but the chambers needed to make the gas a potent treatment are expensive to build and operate. The more doctors who use the technology, the less expensive the equipment and the more affordable for everyone the treatment becomes.

Because hyperbaric oxygen therapy and the other oxygen therapies we will talk about in this book have no side effects for most patients, we can use it as either a primary or an adjunctive treatment for conditions that are considered irreversible, or for which there is currently no effective treatment. There is great potential here for us to see and document patient improvement, or perhaps even outright cures. It broadens our treatment options for many different diseases, particularly because it does not inter-fere with ongoing conventional care.

As a pediatrician, I have been particularly intrigued by the role of HBOT in the treatment of brain injuries in children. In my practice, I have seen great improvement in these injured children and, in some cases, doc-umented reversals of the debilitating symptoms that keep them from lead-ing healthy lives. Brain damage at birth often occurs because of a lack of oxygen, which causes reduced blood flow to the brain and results in the neuromuscular condition known as cerebral palsy. It can freeze or para-lyze a child's limbs, making it impossible for the arms and legs to function properly. Some children are severely uncoordinated, their muscles rigid. Other children require a lifetime of physical, occupational, and speech rehabilitation, with uneven results. Cerebral palsy is actually a general term to describe any brain injury to a developing fetus, or one that hap-pens at the time of delivery or even after birth. It has been my experience that hyperbaric oxygen therapy is very effective in improving these neuro-logical injuries by delivering oxygen directly to children's damaged brains. Additionally, there have recently been some very promising reports coming from physicians using HBOT to treat autism in children. If these reports hold up, it could mean the difference between dependence and independ-ence for the entire family.

Oxygen therapies are not miracle cures. But at the same time, deliver-ing oxygen directly to the cellular level in the human body should be rec-ognized as a way to treat a number of conditions that have not responded fully to the use of other modalities.

Hydrogen peroxide therapy also uses oxygen to heal. Through breath-ing, hydrogen peroxide exists naturally in the body. It works therapeuti-cally by promoting oxidation—the process we defined earlier in which oxygen combines with another substance, changing the composition of both. Hydrogen peroxide is two parts oxygen and two parts hydrogen. Hydrogen peroxide is also an *oxygenator.* In the body, it stimulates a proc-ess we call *oxygenation,* delivering oxygen to the blood and other systems of the body. Toxic reactions can occur in the body when the oxygenation process is not functioning well.

The presence of hydrogen peroxide insures that the immune system functions effectively. In a healthy, balanced body, the granulocytes, the white blood cells that fight infection, produce enough hydrogen peroxide to defend the body from the bacteria, fungi, parasites, and viruses the body takes in. Hydrogen peroxide does other useful work in the body. It is needed to break down carbohydrates, fats, protein, vitamins, and minerals. It regulates hormones, assisting in the production of estrogen, progesterone, and thyroxin, among others. Hydrogen peroxide also helps regulate blood sugar and is important to the production of cellular energy.

Hydrogen peroxide decomposes easily into water and vice versa—water (H_2O) plus oxygen (O_2) becomes hydrogen (H_2O_2). When this happens, it stimulates oxidation, which in turn, increases the body's ability to give more oxygen to the cells. When the body is in a weakened state, unable to produce sufficient hydrogen peroxide, it can be infused into the body to increase its infection-fighting ability, and help the healing process in general.

In my practice, I have used hydrogen peroxide to treat a range of conditions—everything from chronic fatigue immune dysfunction syndrome (CFIDS), migraine headaches, and viral infections to Alzheimer's disease, cancer, heart disease, multiple sclerosis, and rheumatoid arthritis. There are many methods of delivering additional hydrogen peroxide to the body. It all depends on the patient and the illness being treated. Like hyperbaric oxygen therapy, hydrogen peroxide therapy is not new. Introduced into medicine in the late nineteenth century, it has had a rocky history, but because it is a very effective treatment, it has not disappeared. In fact, with the renewed interest in the medical use of oxygen, hydrogen peroxide therapy has also resurfaced as a viable treatment option for physicians.

Ozone is another form of oxygen that is used therapeutically. Ozone takes advantage of both oxidation and oxygenation to do its work. Ozone (O_3) has three oxygen molecules. Because it has one more molecule than oxygen (O_2), it is less stable and easily enters into reactions to oxidize other chemicals. But, during oxidation, the extra oxygen molecule breaks away, leaving a normal oxygen molecule, and increasing the oxygen content of the blood and tissues. That's why ozone therapy is a combination of both oxygenation therapy and oxidation therapy.

Ozone has many practical uses in our society today. Among them, ozone is used to purify drinking water. It is also used to disinfect municipal waste water and clean up polluted lakes and streams. In medicine, ozone kills bacteria and viruses. It can improve blood circulation and act to regulate the immune system. Ozone therapy is known to help greatly in the healing process of troublesome conditions and diseases, such as arthritis, colitis, corneal ulcers, other ulcers, and many others.

Photoluminescence—ultraviolet irradiation of blood (UVIB)—is not typically an oxygen therapy, in that it neither adds oxygen to blood and tissue (oxygenation) nor combines with another substance to change the structure of both (oxidation). However, this process does increase the blood's ability to absorb more oxygen, strengthening the immune system so the body's defenses can organize to get rid of infectious microorganisms. It inhibits the growth of bacteria. UVIB therapy works like this: the blood is taken out of the body, exposed to ultraviolet light, then returned to the body, and when that happens, some remarkable healing takes place. It has a cumulative effect on the body, and each treatment enhances the work of previous treatments. Developed in the 1930s, it was used regularly to treat infections, but with the development of antibiotics, ultraviolet light therapy was pushed to the background, along with other effective, nontoxic treatments that were not as commercially viable. However, as with the other therapies we have discussed, photoluminescence, or ultraviolet irradiation of blood (UVIB), is staging a comeback. In an age of specialization, the fact that it improves the health of almost all patients who have every contemporary disease and condition you can name immediately makes this therapy suspect to the medical establishment. It has been successfully used to enhance, and often cure, people with autoimmune diseases and other illnesses, such as AIDS, allergies, asthma, cancer, influenza, and pneumonia.

As I do with HBOT and hydrogen peroxide therapy, when appropriate, I prescribe UVIB to my patients as part of a complete program of healthcare because I am a very strong believer in their healing powers. The fact that UVIB produces no side effects and has a scientifically recorded history of success, even without medical community approval, should be reason enough to encourage physicians and researchers to try it in cases that do not respond to conventional care. Unfortunately, to date, that has not been the case. In the history of medicine, treatments and procedures that become widely accepted need the approval of conservative institutions, or the power of corporations who can promote a therapy and educate physicians and the public alike. So, when a therapy like UVIB works, as I have seen it work, I believe everyone should have the opportunity to learn about it. In *Oxygen to the Rescue,* you will learn what is required to deliver ultraviolet irradiation of blood to patients. Their progress and response to this therapy will be fully discussed.

With today's interest in alternative therapies, products that can help increase the amount of oxygen the body takes in are very popular. We intuitively sense that our bodies, stressed by the problems of contemporary life, are oxygen-deprived and could use more of it. And products featuring supplemental oxygen as a life-giving and life-supporting key ingredient will be bombarding us before long. In its never-ending search to slow aging and enhance the way our bodies look, the cosmetics industry is already exploring new ways to use oxygen to change the structure of old and deteriorating cells. Oxygenated water is being sold in health food stores. And oxygen bars dispensing pure oxygen in a social atmosphere now exist, particularly in Los Angeles and New York.

From a medical perspective, we know that oxygen can revitalize cells and change cell structure so, theoretically, oxygen could be a key element in the search for the fountain of youth. And perhaps it will be. But we are not there yet. I think it is safe to say that the extra amount of oxygen the body can get—in cosmetic treatments, from drinking bottled water, or having an infusion of supplemental oxygen now and again—is helpful in some small way, but for any real healing to take place, the use of oxygen needs monitoring by a physician within a program of treatment. This does not, however, discount the possibility that commercial entrepreneurs working from a profit motive might add to the growing body of knowledge concerning ways to get more oxygen into our bodies, which is all to the good.

It is quite clear that the destruction of the environment, the deterioration of our air and water supply, our use of chemicals in industry, and the lack of nutrients in our food supply continue to starve our bodies of the oxygen we need. Maintaining and improving our health may soon depend on our ability to supplement the oxygen our bodies can no longer be expected to get naturally. As a complementary physician with a holistic view of the body, I know that oxygen plays a vital role in achieving balance in our bodies, and I consider it a vital part of any individualized treatment program for my patients. It is as important in healing as food and water.

People need to know that oxygen therapies are available to them, not only for the treatment of specific diseases, but also to underline the importance of oxygen in maintaining our health and well-being and in helping to deter the aging process. These are my reasons for writing this book. The practice of complementary medicine demands that we who believe in it are open to new methods. We are attuned to listening to patients and evaluating their complaints and needs. The best of us use whatever treatments we have available to us—both conventional and alternative—to return people to full health. And to do no harm in the process is paramount.

The remarkable scientific and technological achievements of the twentieth century, along with a greater understanding of the nature of disease, have set the stage for new applications of technologies in the twenty-first century. Oxygen therapies are a prime example of this. Introduced in the early years of modern medicine and never given a full opportunity to achieve their promise, they are receiving a long-needed reevaluation of their healing potential. We have a new generation of physicians and researchers who are less cynical and more open to results, and who seem to understand that achieving true healing comes about by dealing with the ills of the whole body/mind. Oxygen, the true breath of life harnessed by us as physicians to use in healing our patients, is a natural direction that becomes more necessary as time goes on. I firmly believe it will become the direction of medicine in the future.

PART ONE

Hyperbaric Oxygen Therapy (HBOT)

Oxygen Therapy Visionaries: A Brief History of Oxygen Therapy

*B*io-oxidative medicine is on the verge of being discovered and, in some cases, rediscovered by both the medical community and the public. But discoveries in the scientific arena do not surface accidentally. They usually happen because a single person champions a theory, either a new one or one that may already exist. In any case, that person's belief in its possibilities is so strong that he or she commits a lifetime, not only to testing it, but also to refining it, fundraising for it, writing about it, and promoting its possibilities. When the theory is a treatment that will help cure illness or improve the health of millions of people, the doctor or researcher is driven by a consuming desire to see the theory applied in practical clinical settings.

Before getting into the specifics of the four oxygen therapies outlined in this book, I'd like to pay my respects to those pioneers who have made it possible for us to heal our patients with treatments that were, and are, far beyond what we learned in medical school.

Dr. Richard A. Neubauer, the medical director of the Ocean Hyperbaric Center in Lauderdale-by-the-Sea in Florida, is one of those visionaries, and I have had the privilege and remarkable experience of knowing him. A physician who received his medical degree from the University of Virginia Medical School, Dr. Neubauer began his career as an internist, and before becoming one of the foremost specialists on hyperbaric oxygen therapy, he held directorships at a number of hospitals where he became even more familiar with the conventional approaches to the treatment of disease.

In 1972, when Dr. Neubauer began to specialize in hyperbaric medicine, he knew his colleagues in the medical profession only accepted ". . .

HBOT for use in wound healing, bone infection, carbon monoxide intoxication, and air emboli or air bubbles in the bloodstream, due to decompression sickness, open-heart surgery, and other sources." He, too, accepted these applications, but Dr. Neubauer gained his reputation as a medical pioneer because of his fierce championing of the more unconventional applications of HBOT widely used in other countries. Such conditions as "coma resulting from head injuries, bruising of the spinal cord, stroke, and neurological disorders, such as multiple sclerosis," among many others, respond very positively to HBOT. Dr. Neubauer's careful documentation of his clinical results and his continued work in this area are responsible for bringing attention to a remarkable treatment that improves the physical lives of patients suffering from these conditions.

Although I had used HBOT in Russia, when I came to this country and learned that very few physicians were even aware of its wide applications, I was both amazed and disturbed. In Russia, we took it for granted that it was highly effective medicine. But here, not only was it considered experimental, but doctors also felt it was dangerous. Only Dr. Neubauer's continuing work and research in this country, against all odds, gave me the confidence to apply this treatment to these additional conditions, even though it was dismissed by the majority of my colleagues.

In addition to his book *Hyperbaric Oxygen Therapy*, Dr. Neubauer has published numerous articles in medical journals and contributed data and case histories to books written by converts to his thinking, and to complementary physicians like myself who apply hyperbaric oxygen therapy on a daily basis in our various practices. Few books exist on the subject, but his, and one by Morton Walker, are considered primary sources of information. I believe it is very important for those of us who, like Richard Neubauer, believe strongly in the possibilities of this treatment to spread the word. It is a remarkable tool for healing, and we are grateful to have this therapy to use for our patients. And they are even more grateful. Dr. Neubauer continues to lecture and hold workshops around the world, offering information, confirming successes, and discussing the reasons for individual failures, to a growing number of doctors, medical journalists, and other professionals who can encourage greater use of the treatment. Ultimately, the fact that HBOT works as treatment where other approaches fail is what will eventually speed its increased use in helping many ill patients return to health.

William Campbell Douglass, M.D., whose committed work on two bio-oxidative treatments—photoluminescence, or ultraviolet irradiation of blood, and hydrogen peroxide therapy—justly defines him as a medical visionary. According to his bio on the cover of his groundbreaking book, *Into the Light,*[1] the only and definitive book on the story of photoluminescence, Dr. Douglass is a crusader. "A vocal opponent of 'business-as-usual medicine,' he has championed patients' rights and physician commitment to wellness for the past two decades."

Dr. Douglass, a graduate of the University of Rochester, the Miami School of Medicine, and the Naval School of Aviation and Space Medicine, is a fourth-generation physician and has been named the National Health Federation's Doctor of the Year. My admiration for his commitment to the application of photoluminescence, or ultraviolet irradiation of blood, and hydrogen peroxide therapy is unending. For an established physician to advocate and apply procedures to patients that are regarded by the medical system as unconventional and experimental is, at best, to put his or her professional reputation on the line. But Dr. Douglass clearly believes that these treatments belong in the mainstream of contemporary medicine instead of being relegated to the fringe, not because they are ineffective, but because of politics and the corporate direction of medicine. The medical establishment would have to deal with the demand that these non-pharmaceutical and nonsurgical oxygen therapies would be considered equivalent to conventional approaches as solutions to disease and illness, and this is difficult for them.

Dr. Douglass is responsible for focusing public attention on photoluminescence and hydrogen peroxide therapy in the last decade. *Into the Light,* his book on the subject, was published in 1992, and since that time, many of us practicing complementary medicine have found it very useful. We have often improved the quality of life for some very sick patients and, in many cases, have even been able to save lives. His book is dedicated to Emmett K. Knott, the father of photoluminescence, to the doctors of Equatorial Africa with whom he worked to help fight HIV/AIDS, and to the Russian doctors, whose continuing work in light therapy has received so little recognition in the West. This, however, is about to change. We can no longer ignore the potential of UVIB and hydrogen peroxide therapy in treating the toxic viruses and bacteria that are global threats to human beings and animals. And we will be able to thank Dr. Douglass for helping us to *use* the light for that.

Hydrogen Peroxide: Medical Miracle by Dr. Douglass is one of the very few books published on hydrogen peroxide therapy. In this book, Dr. Douglass discusses the work of Charles Farr, M.D., Ph.D. Nominated for the Nobel Prize in Medicine in 1993, Dr. Farr is another visionary in the field of bio-oxidative medicine, particularly in the hydrogen peroxide and ozone therapies. One of his contributions was a series of experiments that proved, "contrary to established opinion, (that) oxygen given in the vein (as is done in applying hydrogen peroxide therapy) isn't dissipated in the lungs." Farr also explored combining H_2O_2 therapy with EDTA chelation therapy, and his use of these combined therapies on chronic fatigue syndrome, shingles, and yeast infections is groundbreaking. Additionally, Dr. Farr developed the procedure by which hydrogen peroxide is injected into joints and tissue, and rheumatoid arthritis and other inflammatory arthritis conditions responded quickly to these injections.

These very common conditions trouble thousands of people, and even though conventional drug approaches sometimes alleviate their symptoms, we are dealing with very stubborn problems that often return. In my own clinical work, it has been my experience that, in many cases, H_2O_2 therapy kills these infections, eliminating symptoms completely. Dr. Douglass says, "Many studies within the body and (in) the laboratory have shown that (hydrogen) peroxide will kill bacteria, fungi, parasites, viruses, and (they have) been shown to destroy certain tumors." He goes on to say that "much more work needs to be done, but (hydrogen) peroxide is certainly a universal agent which can *almost always* be tried for an illness, often with great success."

Dr. Kurt W. Donsbach, who founded and runs the Hospital Santa Monica in Mexico, the largest holistic hospital in the world, uses intravenous hydrogen peroxide to treat cancer in patients when conventional cancer treatment has failed. He has also been producing pioneering work, and, in his book *Wholistic Cancer Therapy,*[2] he says there is enough clinical evidence to convince him that intravenous hydrogen peroxide is very valuable in treating cancer because, by increasing the oxygen environment to the cancer cells, it makes them less virulent and in many instances destroys them.

For the past fifty years, we have steadily been fighting cancer, and during that period, researchers and scientists have known that cancer develops in low oxygen environments. Given this knowledge, it seems logical to consider the oxygen therapies I have been discussing as viable treatments, particularly since there are such minimal side effects. Armed with this information, what patient would rather experiment with chemotherapy, with its toxic side effects, than "experiment" with HBOT, hydrogen peroxide, ozone, or photoluminescence first?

Although many individual physicians and researchers have contributed to the knowledge about ozone therapy throughout the centuries, the credit for advancing the cause of medical ozone therapy in these times, primarily since the 1980s, should go to Germany, Russia, and Cuba. As socialist countries, their governments had a pressing interest in developing inexpensive therapies with broad applications. Their governments provide political and financial support for research because they believe, justifiably, that positive results are vital to their societal goals of a healthy population. A policy of universal healthcare demands that the greatest number of people get effective medical care and relief from illnesses as quickly as possible. Therefore, it is only natural that these countries would be interested in oxygen therapies, which work to relieve the symptoms of so many different kinds of diseases, without producing any side effects that also have to be treated.

The documented successes by physicians in these countries are finally getting the recognition they deserve. As with hyperbaric oxygen therapy, hydrogen peroxide therapy, and photoluminescence, the application of ozone in the treatment of patients with chronic illnesses and diseases such as arthritis, cancer, colitis, hepatitis, herpes simplex, and Parkinson's disease have more often than not improved, and sometimes even cured, their conditions.

The definitive book on ozone therapy is *The Use of Ozone in Medicine* by Renate Viebahn, who states the rationale for the interest and research in his preface. "If a substance is indispensable in the preparation of water, it need not (when properly applied) be harmful in the treatment of pathological conditions in the human being."

My personal thanks go to these men and these countries for their development and encouragement of oxygen therapies. Without their work, this book would not have been possible, nor would my patients have the benefits of treatments that, in many instances, were their only possibilities for improvement and cure.

THE GREAT RUSSIAN EXPERIENCE: HOW HYPERBARIC OXYGEN THERAPY BECAME A CORNERSTONE OF RUSSIAN MEDICINE

Dr. Sergei Efuni is a Russian physician who was a pioneer in hyperbaric medicine. Although he is virtually unknown to most American physicians, those of us in complementary medicine have been well aware of the work produced at the State Institute of Hyperbaric Medicine in Moscow while he was its director from 1974–1995. His expertise was considered peerless and his knowledge so extensive that even when he left Russia to live in the United States, he was asked to remain as acting director of the Institute. Dr. Efuni has the highest degrees offered in medicine in his country. Not only is he a medical doctor, but he holds a Ph.D., as well as a Doctor of Science degree, an immensely prestigious and rare achievement, which placed him in an elite circle in the Russian medical and political hierarchy. His colleagues at the Institute relied on him, not just for his mastery of medicine and his administrative expertise, but also for the vast network of connections he could tap. In Russia, as a socialist country, expediting new ideas, getting funding, or easing the way through the bureaucracy was dependent on being able to access the most important members of the medical establishment, government, military, business, and industry.

After completing his studies in Russia, Dr. Efuni went to Holland to work with one of the pioneers of hyperbaric oxygenation in Europe, the Dutch surgeon I. Boerema, who was using HBOT when he operated on patients with valve disease, which allowed him to stop the heart for a longer time and made the operation virtually bloodless. Efuni became fascinated by the extraordinary possibilities of hyperbaric medicine, just in the beginning stages of exploration in Russia, but common in Holland then, as it is to this day—they have more than twenty HBOT centers, a large number for so small a country.

After that, Dr. Efuni came to the United States to explore the work being done at the Department of Hyperbaric Medicine at Duke University in North Carolina, and he became convinced of the importance of establishing an Institute for Hyperbaric Medicine in Moscow. In 1974, Dr. Efuni succeeded in establishing the Institute with funding from the Ministry of the Russian Nuclear Industry. When the ultra-modern facility opened, with him as its director, it became one of the most unique research centers for the study of hyperbaric oxygenation in the world. There were six large multi-place chambers, eight monoplace chambers, and one experimental chamber, staffed by twelve scientists, primarily physiologists, twelve physicians, eight hyperbaric technicians, and twenty on the administrative staff.

The Institute treated 100 patients a day with hyperbaric medicine—alone or in combination with drugs or other therapies—for medical conditions such as acquired heart disease, anaerobic infections including wound infections, cirrhosis of the liver, hypoxic encephalopathy, ischemic heart disease, gastric and peptic ulcers, macular degeneration, major vessel embolism, multiple sclerosis, Parkinson's disease, and shock. A total of sixty conditions were approved for treatment, compared to the thirteen approved in the United States at the time.

At the Institute, HBOT was not used to treat cancer directly, but since hyperbaric oxygen could make a cancerous tumor more sensitive to radiation, its use made it possible to reduce the amount of radiation used in the process. And, since radiation's effect on the body can be dangerous, limiting the amount the body absorbs can only be beneficial.

During his tenure at the Institute, Dr. Efuni witnessed many remarkable recoveries, but one still remains as a definitive example of what HBOT can do. In 1977, he was called in to consult on the case of a twenty-eight-year-old woman in the hospital for a heart valve repair. But before surgery, she experienced an embolic stroke, causing hemiplegia, or paralysis. Her condition was severe. Speechless, she could not move either her arms or legs. Dr. Efuni immediately placed her in a hyperbaric chamber. Within twenty minutes, while still in the chamber, she was able to move her limbs and speak to the members of the staff who were observing her. When the session was completed and the pressure in the chamber was returned to normal, her stroke symptoms also returned. Dr. Efuni recommended two treatments a day for one week, and by the end of that time, she had completely recovered from the effects of the stroke and was able to proceed with her surgery.

His experience over his many years in the field has given those of us who practice complementary medicine in the United States an opportunity to support the work we do with case studies of actual patients, and to learn from them. I had known of Dr. Efuni's work for many years, but we met only two years ago, on the Internet, as he searched for a hyperbaric oxygen facility in the New York City area that could treat a friend with a peptic ulcer. He recognized me from Russian television and called my office. He is now retired, but I feel privileged to have access to his experience and knowledge as one of the world's most prominent authorities on hyperbaric medicine.

I once asked him why he thought American doctors were still so ignorant of this exceptional treatment, and he replied that, as long as American medicine insists on using the double-blind, placebo-controlled research method as the standard for testing new medications and treatments, there will not be a wider acceptance for HBOT. In the double-blind method, two groups of patients and their doctors are kept from knowing which patients in either group are given the placebo. Only after the study is completed are the facts revealed. There is no way to conduct such a study with HBOT because the placebo would have to be air, but air contains oxygen so any study would be invalidated.

Dr. Efuni did point out, however, that the thirteen conditions now approved for HBOT treatment in the United States were *never* subjected to the double-blind studies, which gives the FDA a clear precedent for approving other conditions without the studies.

Dr. Efuni says one of the major reasons that hyperbaric medicine became such an important treatment in Russia (in addition to the facilities devoted entirely to HBOT, every hospital there now has a department of hyperbaric medicine) was that drugs were almost nonexistent. Hyperbaric medicine filled a vacuum. But in the United States, the pharmaceutical companies have the power, and they have little interest in opening themselves up for competition, particularly from a treatment that produces no side effects. (Ironically, however, the issue of drugs' side effects may end up being the wedge into gaining wider availability for HBOT.)

Whether hyperbaric medicine cures people or not isn't the issue. The fact that it can improve patients' health without side effects and can, in many cases, arrest the progress of a disease or a chronic condition is a very attractive feature of HBOT. The demand for this type of treatment is certainly here. It's mainly a question of getting more people to know about it.

The only negative I can see in Americans accepting HBOT is that the treatment takes a great deal of time. The more serious the condition, the longer it takes. There are no shortcuts, and we are a society that wants everything quickly—instant cures, quick fixes. This is not hyperbaric oxygen therapy. People will have to choose between drugs that act quickly, but have side effects (some of them very serious) and HBOT, which demands anywhere from 40 to 200 treatments, plus travel time and cost. In Russia and in Cuba, the treatments are subsidized by the government. In the United States, with no government support and no insurance to cover costs, only those who can pay can have access to treatment.

I believe that the future of HBOT lies in the fact that hyperbaric medicine works so effectively with antibiotics to increase the speed and effectiveness of the healing process. When the pharmaceutical companies begin to realize this, they will want to join forces with us because they will see that, not only is there money to be made, but there are also benefits to be had. It is my hope, and Dr. Efuni's, that one day all medicine in America will be as integrative as it is in Russia.

For now, however, it is important for all of us interested in healing to know that an entire approach to treating disease is not visible in the United States, and we should do everything we can to change that. In Cuba, Japan, the Netherlands, and Russia (among other countries), hyperbaric oxygen therapy is accepted as common treatment and it has the full support of their governments. Why? Because it works!

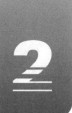

Hyperbaric Oxygen: Reexamining an Old Therapy

*M*ost people have actually heard about hyperbaric oxygen therapy without knowing its technical name: A news organization reports a story on a potential drowning victim saved from death by an infusion of oxygen; a television anchor talks about a family miraculously revived in the hospital after being exposed to carbon monoxide in their home. These lives were most likely saved by the use of hyperbaric oxygen therapy, a simple treatment that forces pure oxygen into the body under pressure for therapeutic purposes.

Hyperbaric oxygen therapy may be one of the most commonly used and yet unknown conventional treatments in medicine today. The reasons for its shadow existence in American medicine is confusing to patients who have benefited from its use and to the physicians who have seen its curative potential at work. Although it has wide application and proven success in treating many contemporary diseases and health conditions, mostly outside the United States, the medical establishment limits its use to fifteen areas, including carbon monoxide poisoning, decompression illness in divers, effects of gas gangrene, and smoke inhalation. The work it accomplishes in these areas is often dramatic and lifesaving, but I believe HBOT's real potential lies above and beyond its conventional uses. This broader arena includes treating the effects of brain injuries, cerebral palsy, encephalopathies, HIV/AIDS, Lyme disease, multiple sclerosis, and stroke.

The history of hyperbaric oxygen therapy goes back at least 300 years when a British physician named Joseph Henshaw first used "compressed air in a specially equipped room called a domicillium."[1] It was his belief that a patient's digestion and respiration could be improved by breathing

23

in pressurized air. But HBOT achieved its real credibility in the diving industry. During the eighteenth and nineteenth centuries, researchers worked to find a way to deliver pressurized oxygen to divers suffering from decompression illness or the bends—a condition that occurs in divers when the nitrogen that accumulates in the bloodstream changes into gas when the deep-sea diver comes up out of the water too quickly. The gas bubbles restrict blood flow and delivery of oxygen to the body. It is very painful. Divers are often unable to stand up straight, which is why the disease is referred to as the bends. When pure oxygen is placed under pressure and forced into the bloodstream, the nitrogen bubbles are displaced and the diver's health slowly returns to normal. The commercial uses for HBOT were not technically developed until 1935, but today it continues to be the primary treatment for diving accidents.

The general public is also unaware of another very common use for HBOT as the treatment of choice for people exposed to carbon monoxide. There are 40,000 emergency-room visits a year in the United States for acute carbon monoxide poisoning. People go to hospitals complaining of symptoms such as dizziness, headaches, memory loss, nausea, vomiting, and even chronic fatigue. A chronic condition may develop when people get exposed to carbon monoxide over time in unsafe work situations or at home. This toxic gas interferes with the blood's ability to carry oxygen through the body. Hemoglobin—the iron-binding protein in red blood cells that normally transports oxygen—is prevented from doing its work by the carbon monoxide. And the result is a low-oxygen environment that threatens the health of the body. HBOT forces out the carbon monoxide and pure oxygen is quickly delivered to the cells.

Countless numbers of New Yorkers were exposed to carbon monoxide during and after the collapse of the Twin Towers on September 11, 2001, and they continued to experience symptoms long after the event— dizziness, fatigue, and headaches, to name just a few—without suspecting the cause was carbon monoxide poisoning.

Many smokers are unaware that when tobacco burns, one of the toxins it produces is carbon monoxide. If they realized they were cutting off oxygen to their cells when they smoked, smokers might have second thoughts about continuing this life-killing process. People who are victims of smoke inhalation from fires take in both carbon monoxide and cyanide. Cyanide poisoning is commonly treated with sodium nitrate, but pure oxygen delivered to the cells under pressure usually helps increase the effectiveness of the antidote. Hyperbaric oxygen therapy displaces any and all toxic gases quickly when fire-induced smoke inhalation occurs. The infusion of pure oxygen can be lifesaving.

People involved in serious car accidents in this country are intimately aware of the importance of hyperbaric oxygen therapy in the treatment of wounds that develop gas gangrene. This painful condition arises in the soft tissues that have been deprived of oxygen due to an injury characterized by blood poisoning, gas, swelling, and tissue death caused by *Clostridium perfringens,* a virulent microbe that thrives in low-oxygen environments. Very few people realize that, although surgery and antibiotics are the major treatments for gas gangrene, the best results are achieved when HBOT works hand in hand with surgery. The oxygen kills the bacteria and limits the production of toxins. This treatment distinguishes between live and dead tissue, and in this way, less surgery needs to be done on seriously injured patients. It is a prime example of how all of us and our healthcare providers need to be aware of the effectiveness of HBOT when used in combination with more conventional approaches to treatment. In the case of gas gangrene, using HBOT can reduce the extent of amputation (and sometimes even the need for it), and increase the survival rate of patients who have severe trauma. Every hospital and emergency room in the country needs to be provided with the technology and equipment to make hyperbaric oxygen therapy available to us when we need it.

The growing interest in HBOT more than fifty years after its initial success is not surprising. In that time, we have become accustomed to its availability; no more efficient, effective methods for treating certain conditions have been developed. Researchers have analyzed the way oxygen under pressure works to heal wounds and destroy bacteria and viruses, and the concept of finding new applications for this tried-and-true approach has intrigued them. Oxygen is, after all, available and free for the taking. If its therapeutic power gets acknowledged in mainstream medicine, its effect on patients will be dramatic. At a time when pharmaceutical treatments and surgical procedures are costing people more than they can afford to pay, oxygen therapies could revolutionize the treatment of many of our most serious physical ailments.

With HBOT, the cost is in the chambers that deliver the oxygen to the patient. The monoplace chamber, large enough for one person, costs between $100,000 and $200,000. The cost of multiplace chambers depends on the number of patients they are designed to accommodate, and can run into hundreds of thousands of dollars. But hospitals are, in fact, not averse to buying expensive equipment if the board believes income can be generated from use of that equipment. For example, magnetic resonance imaging (MRI) scanners are very expensive, more than $1 million to install, and an equal amount to service, but the return on the hospital's investment makes it worthwhile. Used as valuable diagnostic tools, insurance companies will pay for early MRI testing, in order to avoid treatment that would cost even more in the long run. When the demand for HBOT increases—and that is happening, although very slowly—insurance providers will be more inclined to reimburse hospitals.

The ultimate cost of any approach depends on the progress of an illness and the continuing treatments required, particularly if a cure is not effected. HBOT sessions may be more expensive per treatment than a drug, but within a fixed time frame, I know whether it is working or not.

Experts in the field, including Dr. Richard Neubauer, one of the country's foremost HBOT specialists, believe that "the greatest potential benefit of HBOT lies in the fields of cardiology—the study of the function and diseases of the heart—and neurology—dealing with the nervous system, its structure and diseases." My hope is that more of my colleagues will use HBOT so their patients can benefit from its remarkable healing potential. The lack of hyperbaric chambers has not only prevented healing from taking place, but also has caused lives to be lost unnecessarily.

In my practice, I most often prescribe hyperbaric oxygen therapy in combination with other modalities. New patients generally come to me through referrals from current or former patients. By the time they see me, they have often been treated by many other doctors or health practitioners and are still not feeling well. It is common for me to recommend two or three different treatments in addition to HBOT, in the hope that their sum total will result in the improved general health of my patients.

Using Hyperbaric Oxygen Therapy in Conventional Medicine

*H*BOT is the only oxygen therapy approved for use in mainstream medicine. Even though there are restrictions on the specific conditions that can be treated, I feel encouraged by the growing use of HBOT by doctors. However, we should note here that conditions outside the acceptable usage for HBOT are not entitled to insurance coverage, even when the hospital has the equipment in place.

As a physician who practices complementary medicine, I know from experience that HBOT has much wider application in treating disease than is currently recognized. But the success that mainstream physicians have had using hyperbaric oxygen therapy has introduced them to oxygen's healing potential. This leads me to believe that, in the future, other oxygen therapies currently prescribed only as alternative treatments will become mainstream. Today's patients, used to taking more responsibility for their own healthcare, deserve to be given a range of treatment options from which to choose.

HOW DOES HYPERBARIC OXYGEN THERAPY WORK?

A normal body needs between six and eight pounds of oxygen every day. If the bloodstream's delivery of oxygen to any of the cells is blocked, it causes the death of the tissues in the area that is deprived of oxygen. The medical term for this is hypoxia, and it is a serious health issue because any cellular environment in the body that lacks sufficient oxygen is open to disease. There are many reasons why the oxygen we need is not delivered equally to all of the cells in our bodies, and we will talk about the resulting conditions later.

The current terms used in hyperbaric oxygen therapy come from the deep-sea-diving industry. We use this terminology to calculate the amount of pressure needed, even though we primarily treat physical conditions other than the bends with oxygen under pressure.

Understanding the science helps us to understand HBOT treatment better. It is less complicated than it might seem at first. As you may know from your high-school science classes, air pressure has weight because gravity pulls the air around us toward the Earth's center. Above sea level, the higher up in the atmosphere you go, the more the air, or *atmospheric pressure*, decreases. But when a diver goes below the ocean's surface, the atmospheric pressure increases because the water over the diver's head weighs more. The deeper you go, the more the water weighs. This water pressure is called *hydrostatic pressure*. Measuring the total pressure, or *atmospheres absolute* (ATA), you combine the weights of the atmospheric pressure with the hydrostatic pressure, and this is the measurement we use in HBOT. The pressure exerted at sea level is one ATA, which equals 14.7 psi (pounds per square inch). Pressures greater than 1.0 ATA are stated as additional atmospheres absolute, or fractions of them. So when I talk about one hour of HBOT at 1.5 ATA, it means the pressure I am using to treat a patient is one and a half times the average air pressure at sea level.

Hyperbaric oxygen therapy administers pure oxygen to the body at greater than atmospheric pressure, and regardless of the disease or condition to be treated by HBOT, the way it is used is the same. Within a special pressurized oxygen chamber, the patient breathes in pure oxygen, which forces this gas into the tissues of the body. Under normal conditions, only red blood cells carry oxygen—the white blood cells fight infection, and the plasma carries both white and red blood cells. The extra pressure that HBOT exerts on the body allows the oxygen to dissolve into all of the body's fluids. In this way, not just the plasma, but also the lymphatic fluid and the cerebrospinal fluid surrounding the brain and spinal cord, can help carry oxygen throughout the body. This facilitates healing in even the most seriously deprived areas of the body because the extra oxygen improves organ function, allowing the white blood cells to fight infection more efficiently. The body's healing process cannot happen without enough oxygen, and HBOT gets the supplemental oxygen into the tissues quickly, bringing about the energy needed for the body's efficient functioning. Digestion, blood circulation, and breathing are all improved with oxygen.

PREPARING FOR HBOT

There are some simple preparations for those who undergo HBOT. Because we use pure oxygen in this treatment, we take all safety precautions necessary to guard against any fire hazard, although that is a very unlikely possibility. Nevertheless, only 100-percent cotton clothing can be worn during treatment, and we ask women not to wear any makeup, lipstick, lip balm, perfume, hair spray, hair gel, nylon stockings, hairpieces, or wigs. In addition to any of these items, we also ask men not to wear aftershave lotion, and we discourage the use of petroleum jelly or any ointments before treatment. Items such as lighters, matches, cigarettes, jewelry, and watches are not allowed in the chamber, and dentures and partial plates should be removed. We ask that no tobacco products be used during the course of treatment because smoking constricts blood vessels and limits the amount of blood and oxygen that gets delivered to the tissues. Further, treatment may be delayed if there are any symptoms of a cold or the flu— a cough, fever, sore throat, headache, nausea, vomiting, diarrhea, or generalized body aches may delay treatment.

THE TECHNOLOGY OF HYPERBARIC OXYGEN THERAPY

The technical equipment used to deliver pure oxygen is relatively simple. There are two types of specialized chambers—the monoplace and the multiplace. The monoplace can accommodate one person, or an adult and a small child, while as many as thirty people can be treated at one time in a multiplace. The monoplace chamber, a long cylinder with a transparent top, is sealed and pressurized with pure oxygen. Multiplace chambers are rooms pressurized with normal air where those undergoing treatment receive oxygen through a hood or mask.

In a monoplace chamber, the person is either seated or lying comfortably in the unit between sixty minutes and ninety minutes each time. The procedure has three phases:

1. **Compression.** It takes about ten or fifteen minutes for the chamber to become sufficiently pressurized with the pure oxygen.

2. **Treatment.** The pressure is then increased to an appropriate level. During this phase, patients can read, watch television, listen to music, or simply relax.

3. **Decompression.** This is the final phase where the pressure is slowly withdrawn until the level is normal.

When patients are in the treatment phase in an HBOT chamber, they are receiving pure oxygen at the same pressure as a scuba diver who has descended anywhere from sixteen to sixty-six feet underwater. There are three factors we use in calculating an individual session dose of HBOT. First, we use ATA, a diving measure for pressure at a certain number of feet underwater. For example, 2 ATA equals pressure thirty-three feet down; 3 ATA is pressure at sixty-six feet underwater. We treat most conditions at or between 1.5 and 2.0 ATA. Second, depending on the condition being treated, we determine the length of time in the chamber. And third, we determine how often a person needs treatment, the average being a single session, twice a day, five or six days a week for many weeks.

SIDE EFFECTS OF HYPERBARIC OXYGEN THERAPY

The procedure is safe and painless, and there are few, if any, side effects. Some people may feel ear pressure or have their ears pop during compression and decompression, just as they do when an airplane changes altitude. Patients are taught simple methods to equalize inner ear pressure to minimize this effect.

The majority of any HBOT side effects are the result of toxic effects of oxygen. Generally, these side effects are attributed to the reaction between oxygen free radicals and cellular components. Free radicals may inhibit cellular enzymes, damage DNA, and destroy lipid metabolism. This situation can develop when the air pressure is kept higher than 2 ATA for longer than one to two hours without air breaks—a period of ten to fifteen minutes when patients are switched from pressurized oxygen to regular oxygen. Three different organs and systems can be involved:

1. **The pulmonary system.** There are three stages to this: a) tracheabronchitis; b) adult respiratory distress syndrome; c) pulmonary fibrosis. Pulmonary oxygen toxicity can manifest as a pain under the sternum, as tracheabronchitis, or as difficulty in breathing. Also, rarely, a pro-

spective patient might have a condition called pneumothorax, where air is found in the chest cavity surrounding the lungs, or an x-ray will discover an air bubble on the lung. These people are not good candidates for HBOT and their condition should be considered a contraindication to HBOT, not a complication of treatment.

2. **The nervous system.** Only one in 5,000 HBOT patients experiences a seizure, usually after staying in the chamber at 3 ATA for three hours or more. In the very unlikely event of a patient becoming affected by oxygen on the brain, hyperbaric oxygen chambers are equipped with a quick-release mechanism. It is also worth noting that if a seizure does happen to take place, it is harmless and causes no brain damage.

3. **The eyes.** Some HBOT patients experience progressive nearsightedness, which is a reversible phenomenon. Exacerbation of existing cataracts can take place, as can retrolental fibroplasia, which involves changes behind the retina.

The fact that hyperbaric oxygen therapy presents so few side effects makes it an ideal support treatment to other medical procedures, including medication, physical therapy, and surgery.

In considering this therapy, it is important to become aware of its various applications. There are currently thirteen conditions that can be treated in most hospitals, and these are the only ones with assured coverage under most medical insurance policies.

AIR OR GAS EMBOLISM AND HBOT

During surgery or kidney dialysis, or when scuba diving, air or gas bubbles can block an artery or vein, obstructing blood flow to the heart the same way a clot does. Technically, this condition is called air or gas embolism. When it occurs, recompression in a hyperbaric chamber is the recommended treatment.

CARBON MONOXIDE (CO) POISONING AND HBOT

Carbon monoxide poisoning can result from exposure to motor vehicle exhaust or defective gas appliances, or by fires or mining accidents. This, in turn, can cause various neurological disorders or cardiovascular problems, in addition to dizziness, headaches, nausea, vomiting, and flulike symptoms. Infants and children are particularly vulnerable to carbon monoxide poisoning because their developing nervous systems and metabolisms function faster, which makes them more susceptible to the effects of the gas. Studies in pregnant mothers show that, not only does the fetus accumulate higher levels of carbon dioxide, but also the gas is eliminated more slowly than it is in the mother's circulatory system. Oxygen, when under pressure, gets into the bloodstream easier, where it binds with oxygen instead of carbon monoxide. HBOT helps to reduce brain swelling, thereby offsetting the negative effects of breakdown of brain cells caused by carbon monoxide. That is how neurological symptoms are significantly diminished and, in many cases, are completely eliminated.

SMOKING AND HBOT

Treating carbon monoxide poisoning with hyperbaric oxygen therapy is an accepted medical treatment, particularly as it applies to firefighters poisoned by the carbon monoxide present in smoke, or to people affected by faulty gas appliances. They are often rushed into emergency rooms equipped with HBOT chambers. Carbon monoxide poisoning is, however, far more common than any of us realize. Smokers, and those who share their space, may not be aware that carbon monoxide is present in the smoke they inhale and exhale. Low levels of carbon monoxide poisoning in the bodies of most smokers can cause mild to severe symptoms—from dizziness, headaches, and lack of concentration to breathing difficulties, seizures, and even a coma, depending on the concentration of the gas.

Normally, when a nonsmoker inhales, the red blood cells that carry oxygen also carry hemoglobin that binds to the oxygen in the cells and helps release oxygen throughout the body. But when a smoker inhales, the red blood cells take up the carbon dioxide in the smoke, and the body is deprived of oxygen. Lung cancer is the greatest fear of smokers, but in fact, the most serious health hazard smokers face may be the way they are slowly poisoning their lungs, heart, and brain by making it impossible for oxygen to reach the tissues and energize the body. Since it is not categorized as an emergency, treatment is seldom sought. Obviously, however, giving up smoking is a wise health decision, but those who have yet to stop this addiction should know they have a greater need for increased oxygen than the rest of us. It goes without saying that smokers would benefit greatly from HBOT.

SMOKE INHALATION AND HBOT

Smoke inhalation is also treated with HBOT. Increasing the levels of oxygen in the body acts to revive people quickly and greatly reduce the possibility of future ill effects. Smoke inhalation also makes people vulnerable to cyanide poisoning. And treating them with HBOT—in addition to increasing the oxygen in their blood—can also maximize the effectiveness of other antidotes, such as sodium nitrate, the more traditional antidote for cyanide poisoning.

DIMINISHING THE EFFECTS OF RADIATION WITH HBOT

Radiation therapy is widely used for the treatment of cancer, but few people talk about the common side effect of radiation tissue damage. And even fewer people know the advantages of using HBOT to treat this condition, including many physicians who are convinced that the effects of radiation disappear within several months, leaving few, if any, long-term effects in its wake. By increasing the amount of oxygen in the tissues, HBOT can stimulate the skin to form new collagen and new capillaries to bring back full functioning to the tissues. HBOT can also improve the general health of a person undergoing radiation treatments and make them feel better.

The use of radiation after surgery to treat most early stage cancers is common and extends treatment for weeks after the initial diagnosis. Sometimes radiation is used to destroy the tumor itself, but more often, it is used to kill any stray cancer cells that might still exist near the surgery site.

Although it is commonly believed that the effects of clinical radiation dissipate after several months, many patients complain of vague illnesses and discomfort long after treatment has ended. While it is difficult to connect the symptoms with a possible cause, radiation damage—radionecrosis—is a fact. Tissues and organs may be damaged, blood vessels and arteries affected, and even as long as five years after exposure to radiation, the body may not be free from the effects. The radiation reduces oxygen and blood flow. Even though the rays are only targeted to the area under treatment, the entire body feels its effects. The organs begin to function at a less than optimum level, and the immune system becomes sluggish and less able to protect the body against infection. HBOT can go a long way toward restoring balance to the body and preventing vague radiation-related illnesses from surfacing months and years later.

The reason for this is simple. Radiation causes hypoxia, a condition that results when the tissues are deprived of oxygen. When the body is assaulted by radiation, the cells need increased oxygen to come back to life and start healing. HBOT does that. However, as a physician with long experience in treating patients with HBOT, I suggest that it is important to wait several months or a year after the last radiation treatment before beginning with HBOT, in order to avoid stimulating radiation's effect on the body. When seeking help, you have to be careful to choose an experienced hyperbaricist who is familiar with the research on various conditions and diseases, as well as one who understands the equipment and is able to monitor you during treatment. Every person's body is unique and responds to treatment, drugs, and stress—both physical and emotional—in very different ways, so it naturally follows that a full range of results will occur with hyperbaric oxygen therapy as well. Everything is possible, from complete cures or a marked improvement, to a reduction of symptoms, or little or no improvement. Having said that, it is important to repeat that most people respond positively to this therapy, and if, in rare cases, a person's health remains unchanged, there are still few side effects noted.

Radiation can affect soft tissue, including the nervous system, the head and neck, the gastrointestinal or urogenital tracts, and can also cause the bones to weaken and become brittle. Radiation, in fact, has the capacity to destabilize all the structural supports of the body, so it is important to do whatever you can to minimize its potentially catastrophic side effects.

ADDITIONAL USES FOR HBOT

Earlier on, we talked about HBOT for the treatment of gangrene or dead tissue. Wet, or infected, tissue is referred to as gas gangrene. This type of gangrene is caused by a low-oxygen bacteria that rapidly produces deadly toxins that can destroy tissue, cause blood vessels to leak, slow circulation, and even destroy blood. Applied early, hyperbaric oxygen therapy can stop the production of these toxins and slow the pace of the infection. It can also stimulate the formation of new blood vessels. Gangrenous wounds resulting from accidents or trauma, or most particularly from cases of advanced diabetes, often result in amputation of toes, feet, legs, fingers, hands, and arms. Using HBOT as an adjunct to surgery and antibiotics, we can save precious limbs and dramatically improve healing.

When there is severe trauma to bones, soft tissue, nerve cells, or blood vessels, as happens with crush injuries from automobiles or similar accidents, hyperbaric oxygen therapy is a remarkable healer. If severed limbs need to be reattached to the body, HBOT reduces the swelling, helps to restore the vascular function, and aids in conquering infection. Conditions that occur when there is a lack of blood in either tissues or organs, such as compartment syndrome or other acute traumatic ischemia, benefit greatly from the use of HBOT. Compartment syndrome is a condition where the pressure on an artery is so great that it stops the flow of blood, thereby preventing oxygenation of the area. In this case, tissue death, particularly muscle tissue, is the great concern. The sooner we can get oxygen to the area, the greater the chances of tissue recovery are.

The development of hyperbaric oxygen therapy began with researchers trying to find a treatment for decompression sickness. Today, it is still the primary cure for this painful condition that underwater divers occasionally experience. The nitrogen bubbles that accumulate in divers' bloodstreams when they ascend too rapidly are replaced by oxygen under pressure, which relieves the pain and enhances normal breathing.

Problem wounds are those that do not respond to drugs or surgery. Conditions such as diabetic wounds or amputation sites that won't heal can lead to tissue death due to hypoxia, low blood flow, or infection, and the possibility that anaerobic (low-oxygen-environment bacteria) organisms will develop. Again, the quick use of hyperbaric oxygen therapy at the site of the wound begins the healing process immediately.

When a patient with severe anemia cannot receive blood transfusions for medical or religious reasons, the intermittent use of HBOT can be an alternative treatment because it can supply enough oxygen to support the basic metabolic needs of the body's tissues until the red blood cells are restored.

Mainstream medicine recognizes HBOT as an effective adjunct treatment for a condition known as necrotizing soft tissue infection (soft tissue that is dying). Again, the primary treatments for this condition are usually surgery and the use of antibiotics. These infections are often caused by anaerobic and aerobic bacteria existing at the site. The low levels of oxygen, in turn, discourage certain functions of the immune system, and whatever oxygen does exist is depleted. Oxygen under pressure improves the body's healing potential in this case.

When bone marrow and the adjacent bone are infected with bacteria, the condition is called refractory osteomyelitis. Most often the bacteria is a staph infection, and when it doesn't respond to antibiotics or surgery, HBOT is very useful, again as an aid to an aggressive medical and surgical treatment. HBOT can prevent its spread to other parts of the body. It also stimulates the production of new blood vessels, bringing fresh blood, oxygen, and white blood cells to the bone site to fight the infection.

When a person needs skin tissue grafts or flaps (a mass of tissue) transplanted, HBOT is very effective in preserving these tissues. Generally, grafts and flaps come either from the patient's own body, for example, when a vein is taken from a person's leg in order to make a blood vessel for the heart during a coronary bypass, or from a donor when a kidney or heart gets transplanted into a patient. Increasing oxygen to the graft or flap site encourages new blood vessel formation and collagen synthesis to take place. When a large surface of skin needs replacing, administering HBOT in advance of surgery can prepare the area for the new graft to take hold.

Major burn centers know that infection is the leading cause of death in thermal burn injuries. Burns also require prolonged healing time and patients can end up with excessive scarring. It is important to minimize any edemas (tissue swelling). The viable tissue must be preserved and the integrity of the blood vessels must be maintained. Even a brief exposure to HBOT can help to inhibit infections, and when the therapy is applied within the first four hours following the injury, or sooner, the healing potential is maximized. The comedian Richard Pryor is one of the most famous people to recover from third-degree burns because his doctor relied on hyperbaric oxygen therapy. Not only were the burned areas healed, but the unburned parts of his body, from which grafts were taken, were also treated. There is no question that it was a lifesaving procedure for him on every level. He healed completely and continued to perform on stage and television for many years after the accident.

Mainstream medicine has acknowledged an impressive list of conditions and illnesses that respond to HBOT treatment, but this does not guarantee that patients will be treated with HBOT for any of these problems. Many parts of the country simply do not have the equipment, and even if the equipment is available, doctors may not know to apply the treatment. That being the case, you can well imagine that using this tried-and-true therapy for the most recent and most virulent diseases—many the result of harmful environmental and social changes in our society—is even more controversial. However, as you will see in the next chapter, its expanded use is well worth the exploration, investigation, and challenge. Developed in the twentieth century, there are great opportunities for its application in the twenty-first century and beyond. And the need for it becomes more urgent all the time.

Experimental and Innovative Uses for HBOT

I have often wondered why so many of my colleagues working in this profession are reluctant to consider taking advantage of the healing potential of hyperbaric oxygen therapy beyond its most conventional applications. The wider potential for HBOT can make a serious difference in the health of many people who have conditions and diseases that have not responded to conventional treatment. The research is there and the work continues daily around the world, as informed doctors, with their patients' permission, prescribe HBOT for serious diseases such as cancer, cerebral palsy, HIV/AIDS, Lyme disease, and stroke, knowing that the majority of patients will experience few, if any, side effects. While the existing studies have been conducted with small samples, and there have been only a few that followed patients long term, the positive results are there and they demand further investigation. In addition, the testimonials and anecdotal reports are impressive and should arouse the curiosity of those who are serious about healing.

In my personal practice alone, by applying HBOT to a range of conditions and diseases, I have helped my patients achieve remarkable results. Most of the very ill ones have been returned to a sense of well-being. Although it is not always a cure, the treatments very often help to stabilize the condition of those with serious diseases.

A NEW WAY TO TREAT STROKES

Strokes occur when the blood circulation to the brain is cut off. It can happen if an artery is blocked or narrowed, often by a buildup of plaques of cholesterol or other matter on the arterial walls, which, in turn, causes the flow of blood to diminish or stop altogether, a condition known as ischemia. Strokes can also occur when blood clots or emboli develop and cut off circulation, or when there is bleeding in the brain, a condition called cerebral hemorrhage. Often, the body gives us a warning before a stroke, and people experience a transient ischemic attack (TIA), basically a mini-stroke that can last anywhere from a minute or two to a few hours. The important thing to know is that a TIA increases a person's chances of having a serious stroke within five years. Whenever someone has a stroke, mini or otherwise, an area of decay, known as an infarct, develops in the brain. The size of that infarct can predict the possibilities for recovery. Usually, there is an irreparably damaged area at the core, and surrounding that is more tissue that is less affected. Between those two sections and normal tissue is an area known as ischemic penumbra. The cells in this area are often knocked out of commission by the initial stroke and are not functioning, but they are not dead either. HBOT can revive these stunned cells and allow them to resume functioning.

Conventional treatment for strokes usually consists of drugs to relieve the high blood pressure, spasm, and swelling, and surgery to remove any affected tissue, to reduce spasticity (rigid muscles), and to relieve pressure in the brain. Alternative approaches include various herbs, acupuncture, and hands-on therapies, such as massage, cranial sacral therapy, and chelation therapy. But in general, conventional medicine believes that if the body does not recover on its own or respond to the drugs or surgery, then any real recovery from strokes is probably unlikely. HBOT, on the other hand, with its ability to revitalize live, but sleeping, brain neurons by rousing them awake with an infusion of oxygen has managed to show results in people who have not shown improvement for years. Of course, not all stroke patients recover from their disabilities, but in those cases where there is recoverable brain tissue, and where improvement is possible, HBOT can produce results that look like miracles. It all depends upon the size of the ischemic penumbra—the larger the penumbra, the greater the possibility that HBOT can return the stroke patient to normal functioning.

After a stroke occurs, the brain goes through a period of trying to reorganize itself. The ability to do so, by separating out the whole cells and have another area take over the function of that part of the brain that has been damaged, is a critical indicator for recovery. If possible, we apply HBOT immediately after the stroke, and then again after the brain has had a week or so to reorganize itself. Getting oxygen to the affected site helps to decrease swelling and can bring the sleeping cells, the neurons, back to life. Ideally, the sooner HBOT is applied, the more likely it is to be successful. However, according to a March 1990 article in *The Lancet,* nonfunctional neurons can be revitalized even thirteen years after a stroke. Oxygen under pressure can penetrate stroke-affected tissue and increase the amount of oxygen reaching the blood, lymph, and spinal fluid that washes the spinal cord and brain. HBOT causes blood vessels to constrict, which reduces swelling in the brain. It can also soften the rigidity that often develops in a stroke patient's muscles, making physical therapy possible.

Strokes are not yet among the conditions officially approved for HBOT treatment in the United States, even though patients who find out about its potential for healing seek out this therapy and experience vast improvement in their functioning after receiving it. In Germany, it is another story. Stroke patients in Germany regularly receive three-week intensive courses of HBOT, and it is all paid for by their insurance companies.

The case histories of my patients read like mystery stories. Other investigators may have failed to solve the problem, or may not have been aware that the condition being treated was only part of the solution. Treating the whole person often means a more personalized diagnostic process. And some of my most challenging and gratifying cases have been those with a history of mini-strokes or even big-time strokes—cerebral vascular accidents. I usually see these people after their conventional medical treatment is completed. Their physicians have prescribed ongoing medication for maintenance, but there is very little expectation of any more real change in their physical condition, so they continue to live with the effects of the attack and are often depressed and anxious. I have also seen those who have had silent strokes, or experienced symptoms that lasted only a couple of hours, but reported that, within a year or two of the mini-strokes, they developed symptoms such as confusion, memory loss, and even dementia. These stroke-related symptoms appear quite similar to those seen in people with Alzheimer's disease, which—all claims to the contrary—will *not* respond to HBOT.

VASCULAR DEMENTIA

The similarity of symptoms may lead inexperienced practitioners to believe they are treating a person with Alzheimer's disease when in all probability the symptoms stem from a vascular dementia, which *does* respond—very successfully—to HBOT. The clinical features of the two conditions differ, as do the paths of each illness, which is one of many reasons for doing a very careful diagnostic examination.

Vascular dementia, once called arteriosclerotic dementia, is a blockage of the arteries by blood clots, or a thickening and loss of elasticity in the arteries. Some of its symptoms include depression, impaired intellect, loss of focus, memory loss, personality changes, and inappropriate responses to situations and people. Often, people who have a vascular dementia have a history of transient ischemic attacks (TIA), and they occasionally experience short bouts of impaired vision, loss of consciousness, or paralysis. As mentioned above, hyperbaric oxygen therapy, which is very helpful in the treatment of vascular dementia, is not at all effective in treating Alzheimer's disease. So it is very important to take time to discover the true cause of the symptoms before recommending treatment. Physicians tend to be busy and harassed, and often surmise that the symptoms I have described indicate Alzheimer's disease, which is not curable. A person diagnosed this way, who in fact has vascular dementia, wastes many months on prescription drugs and other kinds of treatments that could be more productively spent on a therapy that can produce a cure. The reason for applying HBOT to someone with vascular dementia is that it works better than anything else I know to get oxygen quickly to the brain. When oxygen is forced into the blood cells, the amount that can be absorbed increases, and this leads to the development of new capillaries that can link the arteries and veins. The swelling in the brain decreases, the memory returns, moods stabilize, and the patient can think better and finally feel well enough to return to normal functioning. Very often, using HBOT in conjunction with some of the other oxygen therapies we discuss in this book can greatly help to speed the recovery from vascular dementia.

HBOT AND COMPLEMENTARY APPROACHES

There's no denying the role of conventional medicine in treating an emergency stroke, but after the emergency is over, serious stroke patients generally only improve naturally up to a certain point. To come back to full functional health after a TIA or a cerebral vascular accident (CVA), complementary approaches need to be applied. And to do that, you have to

From Mrs. Zombie to Normal Annie

Annie was an eighty-five-year-old woman who came recommended by a physician in Staten Island familiar with my practice. She was very confused, had a deteriorating memory, and severe osteoporosis. She also had arthritis and had undergone multiple hip and knee replacements. When I met her, she was seeing a neurologist who had discovered evidence of a transient ischemic attack (TIA) after examining her CT scans. She was put on Sinemet, a drug typically used to treat Parkinson's disease, and Aricept, a medication used in an attempt to stabilize Alzheimer's disease, which, in my experience, has not been effective. She was also on antidepressants and multiple other medications.

Annie was accompanied by her daughter, Rachel, who told me she had very little hope that her mother's condition could change, but the recommending doctor thought she would benefit from treatment with me. Annie had very poor communication skills and was vague and hostile. When Rachel pointed out Annie's symptoms to her, Annie denied having them. "My mother is confused," said Rachel. "I am?" asked Annie blankly. I recommended hyperbaric oxygen therapy and with only twenty treatments so far, she has vastly improved. I also put her on chelation therapy, a remarkable treatment that provides exceptional antioxidant effects in the body. It draws heavy metals from the blood by introducing a chelating agent, EDTA (synthetic amino acid ethylene diamine tetraacetic acid), an antioxidant that binds heavy metals and causes them to be eliminated from the body through urine and feces. She has both HBOT and chelation on the same day every forty-eight hours for five days. In this way, we double up on the amount of oxygen reaching her cells.

Annie is very much improved, and her symptoms are less apparent every day. She has been able to cut down on her medications, her confusion is gone, her memory is clearer, and she is free from depression. She still has twenty more treatments of HBOT and chelation to go, in order complete her recovery, but her only real problem now is her knee. Once known in my office as Mrs. Zombie, Annie has really come back to life. She is cheerful, communicative, and alert. And her daughter Rachel, so recently skeptical about the benefits of complementary medicine, is a complete convert. "You have to see Mom to believe that she could be the same person," she tells people.

know that those options are available to you. No one needs to live with the aftereffects of a stroke—minor or major—if HBOT is available to expedite and sustain improvement.

The SPECT (single photon emission computerized tomography) scan is a remarkable imaging system that works in combination with HBOT and is used most commonly in visualizing the brain. For those of us whose medical practices include HBOT and who treat many people with strokes, this is a particularly useful technological tool. It is very effectively used before HBOT to measure the extent and nature of the stroke, and after therapy to analyze the degree of improvement. The process involves injecting the patient with a small amount of radioactive tracer, which moves through the bloodstream to the brain where it binds to active neurons. Then, a special camera takes color pictures of the brain so we can see where the tracer is most in evidence to learn where the active neurons are. SPECT, CAT (computerized axial tomography), CT (computerized tomography), MRI (magnetic resonance imaging), and PET (positron emission tomography) are all technologically sound ways to see inside the body and determine how it is working. CAT and CT scans—elaborate x-rays—were developed to visualize the body's interior structure. MRI uses magnets and radio waves to take pictures of organs and body processes. An MRI scan can document brain changes earlier than a CAT scan. PET is a very expensive imaging process that is capable of measuring both blood flow and brain function in one session. But SPECT is the most effective system to date to measure the brain damage done by a stroke because it points out those areas of the brain that show a potential for recovery. If we compare CAT scans or MRI to a still camera, SPECT is the equivalent of a video camera.

The July 1999 issue of the *Townsend Letter for Doctors and Patients* contained an article coauthored by Dr. Richard A. Neubauer and myself. In this article, "New Frontiers: Anti-Aging Properties of Hyperbaric Oxygen Therapy," we discuss the restoring of brain functioning as "one of the many important goals of anti-aging therapies," and we talk about using the SPECT scan before and after HBOT treatments to document results. As early as the 1970s, Dr. Neubauer put forward the concept that HBOT can help to reactivate the ischemic penumbra, and that symptoms caused by a diminishing oxygen supply of vascular origins can be alleviated, even eliminated, by using HBOT. But, again, cases of Alzheimer's disease do not respond to this treatment.

We have presented three cases to support the application of HBOT to patients with conditions that had vascular origins. There was a seventy-year-old woman who began to notice "periods of confusion, forgetfulness, and agitation and had reached the point where she was unable to drive her car or live alone." A SPECT scan showed that HBOT could help improve her condition. She received a total of thirty-three treatments. After thirteen sessions, there was improvement, and by the time she had received twenty, she was back to living a normal lifestyle. After two and a half years, she has had three maintenance HBOT treatments and is still doing very well.

We also treated a man who had suffered a stroke and had been complaining of dizziness, stiffness, and neck pains, as well as memory loss, for two and a half months. After ten HBOT treatments of one hour each at 1.5 ATA, all his symptoms were improved and "he felt much stronger, with increased energy." A follow-up SPECT scan was conducted after ten treatments, and it confirmed significant improvement from the original base scan taken when he first came in for consultation.

The third case was a personal one for Dr. Neubauer. After his bright and alert seventy-two-year-old secretary retired, her daughter called saying that her mother was moving in with her because she was "confused, disoriented, dizzy, and weak." A SPECT scan was taken, and she was given four hyperbaric oxygen treatments for one hour each at 1.5 ATA, followed by a repeat SPECT scan. "The results were dramatic," according to Dr. Neubauer. His former secretary was able to return to living on her own, driving her car, and taking care of all her own personal affairs.

Using HBOT for anti-aging purposes is becoming more and more important to a graying world population. It could make a major difference toward the goal of keeping older women and men active, vital, and able to continue making contributions to society as they move into their eighties, nineties, and even hundreds. SPECT scans before and after hyperbaric oxygen therapy treatments can offer scientific documentation of the efficiency of this underutilized treatment. We hope this book will help to broaden the options for making this treatment available to everyone who is in need of help.

WHY HBOT TREATMENTS MAY NOT BE CONTINUED

There are three possible reasons why some who begin HBOT do not continue treatment. I see many people who come for various neurological disorders. In order to see real improvement, it is often necessary to have at least 80 to 100 treatments. Many people have neither the patience to see a long course of treatment through to success, nor the belief that they will feel sufficiently better if they stay the course. Secondly, a family runs out of financing. And finally, also related to money, the person realizes his or her family is covering the costs and doesn't want to further burden them or feel obligated. And those who are usually treated in a conventional medical setting generally believe that insurance covers all medical expenses. It doesn't. Since insurance companies will only reimburse patients for HBOT treatment of *approved* conditions, the cost of this treatment for any unapproved diseases or conditions must be absorbed by the patients themselves. Oxygen, the only ingredient in the treatment, is free, but the delivery system continues to be expensive. Hyperbaric oxygen chambers cost money to construct and maintain. (In Russia, the manufacture of hyperbaric oxygen chambers is big business, bringing down the cost considerably, but in the United States, without FDA support, HBOT chambers are very expensive to purchase.) Magnetic resonance imaging (MRI) equipment is also expensive, but it is considered a valuable diagnostic tool for doctors, so the demand drives hospitals to make it available. The costs for its construction and purchase are charged to the patient, and the sessions are paid for by insurance; consequently, every major hospital has one. When hyperbaric oxygen therapy becomes more widely prescribed, insurance companies will also pay for those treatments, which will, in turn, increase the numbers of chambers available for use. The demand for the chambers, however, will not increase as long as physicians and researchers look to the pharmaceutical companies exclusively to provide the research and treatment of illness. The pharmaceutical companies have other priorities for their research funds, particularly since oxygen cannot be packaged as an over-the-counter product. In countries where these drug companies have less influence, HBOT is used widely, and the benefits to patients—not the least of which is no side effects—are many.

It is frustrating to me as a doctor not to be able to see the full measure of improvement possible in my patients just because of financial restraints. But I realize that, in neurological cases where HBOT is particularly useful, patients are pleased with even a 20 or 30 percent improvement because conventional means are unlikely to produce even so much as a 1 percent improvement after the initial treatment is completed.

Hyperbaric oxygen therapy is the only existing treatment method that can improve common symptoms associated with neurological disorders such as brain dysfunction, physical disabilities, and strokes. Most mainstream doctors believe that these symptoms are conditions their patients must learn to accept. In our field, we know better.

It is even more frustrating to know how very few patients come to me directly after a stroke. People do not realize that, with conventional therapy, they can only improve up to a certain level, whereas HBOT can help them continue to improve. Very often, they can be back to living normal lives within a year. I usually see patients two or three, or even twelve years post-stroke. Even then they get better, sometimes miraculously, but I could have saved them years of disability. The good news is that, even if you stop treatment, when you come back, improvement is still possible. The effects of HBOT are cumulative.

SPREADING THE WORD ABOUT OXYGEN THERAPY

My only solution as a physician who has seen the benefits of HBOT in treating patients is to get the word out about the potential of this and the other forms of oxygen therapy we talk about in this book. That is beginning to happen, although at a slower pace than I would like. For those of us who know the value of a natural approach to healing, using oxygen as a treatment makes perfect sense. What could be more natural than oxygen? Harmful low-oxygen environments within the body are known to be breeding grounds for the development of diseases, particularly cancer, so finding ways to bring oxygen to those parts of the body in order to begin healing is a logical direction. It is my hope that books like this will stimulate interest in HBOT and give you the confidence to pursue treatment if and when you need it. If you want information for yourself or a member of your family, or if you are a physician who needs and wants an effective treatment to recommend when others have failed, I urge you to investigate this road less traveled. I have been as impressed by the results of HBOT as I am by the marvels of new medical technology.

I have treated many people with arterial vascular disease, chronic fatigue syndrome, comas, diabetic wounds, encephalopathies, multiple sclerosis, and ulcers, even a few with fibromyalgia—chronic pain in the fibrous tissues of muscles, ligaments, and tendons. HBOT figures strongly in my recommended treatments for many of them; however, as a com-

No Chance for Change

Sam came to see me to humor his wife, Lilia, who had heard about me through the Russian community grapevine in greater New York City. "She's a pain in the neck," Sam complained, "always nagging. I'm only here to shut her up. I know you mean well, doc," he said, "but I've been to a lot of doctors and I'm getting used to being this way." Sam was not in good shape when he arrived at my office for the first time. He had severe balance problems and therefore couldn't walk without a cane or walker. His speech was slurred and his memory had been seriously affected by a stroke that had attacked his cerebellum. Once a very physical person, when Sam came out of his coma, he was no longer independent. I recommended hyperbaric oxygen therapy, and Sam, humoring both me and his wife, replied, "Anything you say, Dr. Yutsis." But after only five HBOT treatments at 1.5 ATA, he noticed a difference in his body, particularly in his physical coordination and balance. It gave him hope and more confidence that, if he continued the treatments, his symptoms would be much improved. After twenty treatments, he no longer needed the walker and used his cane less often. He then received twenty-five more treatments with 1.75 ATA, a little more pressure, and the results were remarkable. His balance was completely restored, and he no longer needed his cane at all. Sam admitted that all his wife's nagging had paid off. From having no hope for recovery, he's now 100 percent back to his former self.

plementary physician, you learn not to be rigid about any single method, but instead to draw from all sources of treatment. A few years ago, I had an exceptionally interesting case. A woman suffering from both chronic fatigue and fibromyalgia for fourteen years came to me specifically for hyperbaric oxygen therapy. We tried for a number of weeks, but in her case, it was not the right treatment. It happens sometimes. She was clearly disappointed and in pain, so the search began for a treatment that would help her feel better. She wanted to do it, and of course, I knew we would eventually come up with the right combination. I put her on hydrogen peroxide therapy, chelation therapy, and acupuncture, and she improved 100 percent.

We don't rest until we get to the root of the problem. Complementary physicians are also fortunate to have access to all the conventional testing results, in addition to our own tests, so we get a complete picture of a person's health. We are in an era of healthcare where doctors push patients out every ten minutes, not because they want to, but because the system demands it. In our field, however, we will take the time to figure out what is really happening in a person's body. Forty-five minutes, an hour, whatever it takes, we explore together as doctor and patient. It's why we are successful, but today this very sensible approach is considered unconventional.

Getting Beyond Survival

Joe was only thirty-five years old when he had a hemorrhagic stroke, a cerebrovascular accident (CVA), while on his job as a police officer. Although he was given very little chance of survival, a clot (hematoma) was removed from the left temporal region of his brain, leaving him alive but seriously impaired. His sister, who listened regularly to my radio show, made an appointment for Joe to see me and accompanied him to my office. During his first visit, it became clear that he had sensory aphasia—he understood what was being said to him, but didn't know that what he answered was incomprehensible. He couldn't connect the information he was receiving with the information he needed to provide in order to be understood. He dragged his feet when he walked and one eye was closed from the stroke. He had heart problems, and it was no surprise that he was also very depressed. Joe had a nine-year-old son who lived with his ex-wife, but even though he and his son saw each other regularly, Joe was uncommunicative and seemingly uninterested in having a real relationship with the child.

He had 125 HBOT treatments in all, coming every day, five days a week—forty treatments at 1.5 ATA and eighty-five treatments at 1.75 ATA. After about sixty treatments, he began taking an interest in his son, talking to him and even playing baseball with him. One surprising fact about HBOT is that the oxygen affects a person's mental acuity first. The speech and thinking skills improve before we observe any change in motor functions. Joe's depression had lifted, and although his speech was not always clear, he could communicate and make himself understood. When last I saw him, he was able to say, "Dr. Yutsis is a very good doctor."

FROM THEORY TO PRACTICE:
HBOT AND MULTIPLE SCLEROSIS

The causes of multiple sclerosis (MS) have been explored for many years. One theory is that MS is caused by a virus, but evidence of there being a true virus has not yet been proven. Another theory speculates that the cause is an autoimmune dysfunction and the immune system is responsible for attacking the nerves and stripping the myelin covering that insulates them. Without the myelin sheath, the nerves can't conduct impulses efficiently, and eventually a short circuit develops. There are those who believe MS is caused by environmental factors, or that blood circulation in the brain is arrested by fat particles. And then there are theories that metals, such as mercury, silver, or copper—either the result of dental fillings or factors in a work environment—act in a toxic way in the body, causing MS to develop. None of these theories has produced any positive results. Regardless of cause, however, drug therapies are used to treat the symptoms and to try and slow the progression of the disease, but there are almost always side effects.

HBOT is the only treatment I know of that helps relieve MS symptoms without producing any side effects. And it works over time. Dr. Richard Neubauer and Dr. Sheldon Gottlieb have developed a theory based on their clinical observations and their research that holds that MS is caused by a lack of oxygen.

In *Hyperbaric Oxygen Therapy*, Dr. Neubauer and Dr. Morton Walker explain that MS is a wound in the central nervous system that arises when blood pressure within the brain and spinal cord becomes elevated and remains elevated for a prolonged period of time. When any blood vessels are damaged, they produce changes within the nerve tissue, as in strokes, and this results in a lack of oxygen, or hypoxia. But in multiple sclerosis, this oxygen-deprived environment leads to the destruction of the nerve fibers' myelin sheaths, and to secondary damage associated with the immune system. In the last twenty years, a number of controlled clinical trials using hyperbaric oxygen therapy have been conducted[1] by physicians and researchers in many countries, and the results show definite improvement in MS symptoms. For example, as stated in *Hyperbaric Oxygen Therapy*, "In 1984, Dr. Neubauer learned that more than 10,000 people in fourteen countries had been treated for MS with HBOT. He found that 70 percent of those tested showed improvement in their brain and bowel-bladder function, and had a lessening of muscular spasticity and other symptoms brought on by the disease. There was also a marked absence of deterioration and few relapses among those who participated in a periodic HBOT booster program."

This treatment for MS is, in my opinion, the best we in complementary medicine have to offer until a complete cure is discovered. Symptoms are improved, and there are no side effects. Because we are dealing with a disease whose symptoms are debilitating and progressive, a treatment that can immediately improve the quality of life is certainly one a person should consider. Drugs may stave off deterioration for a while, but not without side effects. And HBOT, when combined with massage, occupational therapy, psychotherapy, and speech therapy, can be the centerpiece for a health program designed to encourage full participation in work and life.

A ROLE FOR HBOT IN THE TREATMENT OF HIV/AIDS

Human immunodeficiency virus (HIV) is a complicated and deadly disease that is transmitted from an infected person to another through sex or contact with infected bodily fluids. HIV mainly affects the immune system and has been known to remain in the body for many years, showing few, if any, symptoms. The potential for HIV to escalate into acquired immune deficiency syndrome (AIDS) is always present. Because each of our bodies is different, however, it is difficult to know when, or even if, full-blown AIDS will develop in an individual.

Our immune system is a strong and powerful deterrent to the spread of any disease. And when faced with HIV cell replication, it marshals its forces quickly, but over time, its ability to shore up its immune function and to continue protecting the body lessens. When that happens, various infections and diseases attack the body. To date, the treatment against the spread of HIV/AIDS has been primarily pharmaceutical. A number of drugs are used and more are continually being tested to slow the progress of the disease. AIDS is a difficult enemy because it is not a singular one; it is a combination of, not only immune dysfunction, but also infections, malignancies, and physical changes that assault the body with varying degrees of success. Unlike other life-threatening diseases, researchers are faced with a disease that has no predictable pattern of behavior. We know so much and yet it is still a mystery why some people are more vulnerable to the host of infections and symptoms of AIDS than others.

What we have learned, however, is that even though we have not yet found a cure for HIV/AIDS, we can stabilize it by using a multidisciplinary approach. And, while certain drugs used over a long period of time may lose their effectiveness in an individual, HBOT can be used as continuing treatment. For example, according to Michelle Reillo in her book, *AIDS Under Pressure,* pneumocystis carinii pneumonia (PCP), an infection that moves quickly and is life-threatening because of its ability to severely suppress the immune system, can be managed if drugs like Dapsone, Bactrim, Benadryl, and Aerosolized Pentamidine are used along with hyperbaric oxygen therapy. For people who want in-depth information on the use of HBOT to treat HIV/AIDS, I highly recommend this book. It is quite technical, but worth investigating if you or a member of your family has been diagnosed with the disease.

As a registered nurse and a principal investigator on many AIDS research studies, Ms. Reillo has witnessed HBOT's possibilities for helping those with the disease maintain a decent quality of life. She cites the case of a twenty-six-year-old woman with AIDS who "presented with acute PCP following a bacterial pneumonitis," and who had already been "receiving ongoing HBOT three times per week for three years, with a six month hiatus because of a demanding employment schedule." And this was in addition to a complicated drug-treatment program. The woman tolerated the multiple drugs with varying degrees of success, but the application of HBOT sustained her in the PCP crisis, and the debilitating symptoms, such as fatigue, fever, and shortness of breath, were resolved. On the tenth day after the infection set in, she "returned to the gymnasium, walking one-half mile and lifting weights, with progressive improvement to running by day seventeen."[2]

In her book, Ms. Reillo makes a strong case for the use of HBOT along with medications, if they can be tolerated, in the treatment of HIV/AIDS-related cytomegalovirus, dementia, retinal detachment or other eye problems, skin conditions (psoriasis or eczema), and tuberculosis. The oxygen therapy appears to "slow the progression of the disease by enhancing immune function and slowing viral production."

THE HIDDEN CONSEQUENCES OF LYME DISEASE

Carried by the Ixodes family of ticks—of which the deer tick is most familiar—Lyme disease was first discovered in Old Lyme, Connecticut. Because its initial victims were children who complained of a rash followed by joint pains, doctors in the area thought it might be a form of juvenile arthritis. Lyme disease turned out not to be a children's disease, but one that affects people of all ages, particularly in the spring, summer, and early fall when more time is spent outdoors in low grassy and wooded areas. It is most prevalent in the northeast and upper midwest, but has also been found in other parts of the United States and is similar to a tick-borne disease that has been in Europe for many years.

The spirochete microorganism that causes Lyme disease lives on small animals, particularly mice. The deer tick, a tiny insect about the size of a sesame seed, picks it up from the animals and then passes it on to us in a minute tick bite, which can be easily overlooked. The first indication of any infection is a reddish skin rash that develops around the bite and usually lasts from a few days to a month before disappearing. Those with visible symptoms are the lucky ones, however, because more than 25 percent of those infected never develop a rash and may never know they have the disease until they later develop far more serious symptoms.

Lyme disease is difficult to identify because the symptoms are so similar to other diseases. People can develop nervous system disorders, such as meningitis or encephalitis, or simply become confused and emotionally distressed, and experience memory loss. They might begin to develop arthritis or other joint problems, constant headaches, fevers, and muscle pains, or they might become physically exhausted. But with Lyme disease, even blood tests are not always reliable. A person exhibiting symptoms may not test positive the first time around, or someone with no symptoms may continue to test positive for years. If it is difficult to identify Lyme disease, it is even more difficult to treat. If you catch it early and treat it early with a full three-week course of antibiotics, that usually takes care of the problem and cures the disease. Doxycycline, tetracycline, amoxicillin, or Flagyl (metronidazole) are often used to treat adults. Children are treated with amoxicillin, erythromycin, or penicillin G.

The fact that Lyme disease is often not identified early means that, by the time antibiotics are used, the Lyme spirochete is protected by the body against the medication. Even stronger intravenous antibiotics may not fully destroy the spirochete, and people have been known to live for years with symptoms that cause serious damage to their bodies. Those of us who use HBOT as treatment believe it would be effective in treating Lyme

disease because oxygen under pressure as therapy increases the effectiveness of antibiotics and speeds the healing process of all infections, but
clearly more research is needed.

According to preliminary studies reported in *The Lancet* and *The British Medical Journal,* oxygen under pressure, HBOT, appears to attack the
Lyme spirochete directly by forcing oxygen into the body's cells. In their
book, *Hyperbaric Oxygen Therapy,*[3] Dr. Neubauer and Morton Walker cite a
Texas A&M University pilot study on treating Lyme disease with HBOT.
The experiment, conducted by Dr. William Fife and Dr. Donald Freeman,
did not produce definitive results, but did show some degree of improvement in all forty people who participated in the study. They were treated
with HBOT, at 2.36 atmospheres absolute, one to two times a day, five
days a week for one to four weeks. It is reported that all forty developed a
Jarisch-Herxheimer reaction, a sudden passing fever, which is the same
reaction that occurs during any aggressive antibiotic treatment for Lyme
disease. Some felt relief from their symptoms during treatment; others
did not, but reported improvement after HBOT was over. The kinds of
improvements noted were cessation of pain, increased energy, mental
acuity, and relief from anxiety and depression. Some still suffered minor
symptoms, but with HBOT, the symptoms were strongly diminished.

Treating Lyme disease with HBOT makes good sense, particularly if
the disease is discovered late and seems resistant to antibiotics. There is
nothing to lose by trying the therapy, and there is always the prospect of a
successful return to normal health. That is, in fact, also true about treating infections caused by streptococci bacteria. Leprosy is also a bacterial
infection. Although, there are presently no studies or standardized treatment programs for dealing with these various infections, those of us who
believe in the benefits of HBOT know that treating *any* infection with oxygen under pressure will improve a patient's health and, in some cases, will
bring about complete cures with no side effects. We've seen it happen, and
for those who have experienced drug reactions, or are living with symptoms caused by some very recalcitrant bacteria and viruses, HBOT and
other oxygen therapies may be the only known alternative.

TREATING ISCHEMIC ENCEPHALOPATHY AND GETTING RESULTS

The long and complicated-sounding medical term "ischemic encephalopathy" simply refers to abnormal brain function due to an insufficient flow of blood and oxygen to the brain, whatever the cause. As a pediatrician, I have sometimes seen babies or young children show signs of encephalopathy after a birth trauma, such as a cord wrapped around the neck, or other problems that arose during delivery. Also, babies with shaken baby syndrome, or children who have been battered or are involved in automobile accidents, can experience ischemic encephalopathy. In a baby, symptoms such as abnormal activity, seizures, not breathing normally, or producing too little or too much urine need to be monitored carefully for signs of brain dysfunction.

The Ocean Hyperbaric Center, directed by Dr. Richard Neubauer, cites case histories of children with neurological damage given HBOT treatments, either at the time of injury or even several years later, which show strong evidence of improvement in all cases after the oxygen under pressure is applied. After as few as twenty-one treatments, one three-year-old boy who had previously not been able to speak or function normally sat up straight, made new sounds, held a cup in his hands, and was generally alert and aware of his surroundings. And his case is not unusual, except that he is one of the fortunate children to have had the advantage of being treated in a facility equipped to apply hyperbaric oxygen therapy.

The story of Eric is not untypical of the kinds of brain damage cases we see on a regular basis. At two and a half, Eric nearly drowned after hitting his head when he fell into a swimming pool. His parents had no idea how long he was underwater, but after he was rescued, they were told that, not only would Eric be blind, he would also remain in a vegetative state for the rest of his life. After only three treatments with HBOT, however, Eric began moving. He tried to speak and was noticeably agitated when he was angry. After sixteen treatments, he could cry, and after only ten more treatments, Eric smiled and laughed. He was very alert, slept well, and even laughed when he was dreaming. With each treatment, his eye contact improved, and it became obvious that he was not blind. Eric has now received 199 treatments and he not only sees, but speaks two languages, eats and drinks normally, stands alone, and can even take a few steps.

In 1996, Dr. Richard Neubauer, Dr. Henry Pevsner, and Sheldon F. Gottlieb, Ph.D., presented a paper in Milan, Italy, summarizing eight case histories of eight- to twelve-year-old children with severe ischemic encephalopathy. The causes varied from lack of oxygen *in utero,* near drowning, and near fatal hypoglycemia to carbon monoxide and natural gas poisoning. In all cases, "positive effects of hyperbaric oxygen therapy were observed." Mental and physical improvements were noted in each of those treated, leading the doctors to conclude that HBOT can be used, not only in the late stages, but also as primary therapy in the early treatment of all of the conditions causing ischemic encephalopathy.[4]

In adults, the use of radiation over extended periods of time can produce side effects that are not always acknowledged by conventional medicine. In addition to fatigue, lack of focus, and memory problems, more severe side effects can occur. For example, when the brain or spinal cord are irradiated, there is a possibility of encephalopathy damaging the fragile capillaries. Blood clots can form and not only reduce the flow of blood, but also seriously reduce the amount of oxygen in the tissues. Although not numerous, there have been a few studies showing improvement when hyperbaric oxygen therapy is used in combination with drug therapy, particularly the vasodilators that help open blood vessels. Even in late-stage radiation-induced brain disease, improvement with HBOT is noted in all cases, although the degree varies from patient to patient. To make the point again, by bringing oxygen under pressure to the site of injury or blockage, HBOT can more often than not increase the level of improvement in the patient's condition, leading to the inevitable conclusion that this therapy is one of the most effective ways to return full functioning to the brain.

MINIMIZING THE EFFECTS
OF TRAUMATIC BRAIN INJURY

Head injuries are particularly dangerous and require careful monitoring by physicians to determine the degree to which the brain swells and whether there is a potential for brain damage. When the brain swells, blood supply is cut off and cellular waste products accumulate, which can cause a person to lose consciousness and even fall into a coma. According to the Centers for Disease Control (CDC), in 1995–1996, a million people with traumatic brain injury were treated and released from hospital emergency rooms, 230,000 people were hospitalized and survived, and another 50,000 people died from their injuries. It is evident that there is a real need to find ways to prevent these injuries and then to find better ways to treat their aftereffects, which include impaired concentration and memory, mood changes, and diminished physical strength, coordination, and balance. In some cases, tactile sensation and vision are affected as well, and for many, these symptoms can last a lifetime.

Hyperbaric oxygen therapy has been particularly useful in the treatment of traumatic brain injuries. Whether the patient's condition is minor or serious, more oxygen to the brain can only help, and in the worst-case scenarios, when a patient falls into a deep state of unconsciousness, the immediate application of HBOT can help prevent permanent damage. Oxygen gets forced into the blood plasma, which doesn't normally carry oxygen, and infuses the cerebrospinal fluid around the brain, reaching areas that are inaccessible, due to the trauma, to the red blood cells, which normally carry oxygen through the body. HBOT has the capacity to stabilize and repair the cells surrounding the brain and, in doing so, allows the blood/brain barrier to continue its work of protecting the brain from toxic elements.

The extra oxygen can be essential in awakening dormant cells in the penumbra, the area between the damaged and healthy parts of the brain we discussed earlier. It can restore patients to consciousness, help prevent speech loss or paralysis, or even eliminate the possibility of permanent brain damage. Hyperbaric oxygen therapy should be standard emergency care for head injuries, but most trauma centers are either not equipped to do it or do not realize that HBOT can be their most valuable asset in returning brain-injury patients to normal functioning.

Medically, the benefits of HBOT in the treatment of brain injuries include an increase in the amount of oxygen dissolved in blood plasma, an improvement in both the metabolism and utilization of glucose in the affected brain regions, and a serious reduction of pressure on the brain. A randomized one-year study followed a group of 168 people with severe head trauma who were treated with or without hyperbaric oxygen therapy. Thirty-two percent of those treated with HBOT survived, while only 17 percent of the patients *not* treated with HBOT lived. In order to achieve the best results from HBOT, the treatment should be applied as quickly as possible after the trauma occurs. However, since many do not find out about HBOT for years after their traumas, they should know that, even then, HBOT treatments can lead to an improvement in their ability to function.

In Russia, regular studies on the effects of hyperbaric oxygen therapy on cerebrovascular disorders are conducted, as they were when I spent time there as a young physician. They continue to refine their methods, experimenting with changes of ATA to gain maximum improvement in conditions due to brain, and other, injuries. This research has been of great value to our practice in this country where there is limited acceptance of HBOT as a valid treatment by establishment medicine. As recently as 1997, the Russian Medical University in Moscow was in the process of developing a new method for treating cerebral vascular disorder with minimum higher-pressure doses of an oxygen/air mixture.[5] The method, deemed safe and effective, was able to restore cerebral brain function, metabolize energy, and eliminate oxidative stress. Research like this from other countries—only a few institutions in the United States conduct research privately, without government support—allows us to increase our ability to help our patients physically improve beyond their current conditions. Most conventional doctors believe that after initial treatment, their role is to help patients adjust to their inevitable disabilities. It is a major difference in our medical philosophies.

LIMITING THE LONG-TERM EFFECTS
OF CEREBRAL PALSY

Any abnormality in motor control caused by injuries to a child's brain *in utero,* during birth, or even in the first few months after birth, is referred to as cerebral palsy. Every year, as many as 5,000 babies and children are diagnosed with this disorder, so it has become one of the more common chronic problems in children's health.

Cerebral palsy is difficult to diagnose in the first few months of a child's life because the physical symptoms common to the disorder—muscle weakness, neurological disorders, spasticity, and rigidity of muscles—are not easily recognized early on in babies. But as the child grows older, the physical problems become more apparent, and range from mild to severe. Cerebral palsy is not curable, but even in conventional medicine, getting the right therapy can help diminish the impact of symptoms. Conventional treatment consists of physical therapy to help with problems of movement and posture; occupational therapy that focuses on helping a child develop hand functions, primarily for eating; speech therapy; prescribing hearing aids, eye glasses, and medication (mostly muscle relaxants and anticonvulsants to reduce seizures); and, in severe cases, a recommendation of joint surgery as a way of repositioning arms and legs to operate more normally.

Spastic cerebral palsy is the most common type of this disorder. It affects 70 to 80 percent of the children with the condition, and is defined by muscles that are stiff and permanently contracted, resulting in an awkward and uneven gait or movement pattern. The spasticity probably occurs because the myelin sheaths covering the nerve fibers, which exist to speed up the process of transmitting nerve impulses, fail to develop properly. Normally, the myelination process starts about a month or so before birth and is completed by the time a child is about two years old. If there is abnormal swelling in the mid-brain, the cells that form the myelin sheath die and the nerve fibers are exposed. As this occurs, the fibers deteriorate and spasticity develops.[6]

There are other forms of palsy as well, categorized by different movement disorders, but beyond the physical disabilities caused by the brain injury, there are also medical problems for all the children affected. Almost half of them are epileptic or experience seizures. There may also be mental disabilities, although a large percentage—at least one-third—are intellectually normal. The rest have impairments that range from mild to severe. Seeing and hearing are sometimes affected because eye muscles are not aligned, and the hearing mechanism is not developed. Some children do not grow or develop normally, and others struggle with an impaired ability to respond to touch or pain sensations.

Hyperbaric oxygen therapy, in combination with the regular therapy discussed above, has shown great promise in treating cerebral palsy, whether in children or adults. As with other brain injuries where some nerve cells in the brain are permanently destroyed, there are other cells that may simply be dormant because they are deprived of oxygen due to a decrease in the blood flow. When high oxygen levels are applied under pressure, these cells have the capacity to awaken, and this increases their ability to recover. With cerebral palsy, there can be a reduction in some or all of its symptoms in most. However, how much improvement an individual can make depends on a variety of factors, primarily the amount of permanent damage done to the brain. In our diagnostic process with cerebral-palsy children, we have found that SPECT is particularly useful.

A case report on identical twins by Philip James of the Wolfson Hyperbaric Medicine Unit at the Ninewells Medical College provides a view of HBOT in action to help slow the progress of cerebral palsy when applied early. The children were delivered prematurely, at seven and a half months, by cesarean section. On the third day after their birth, ultrasound scanning showed hemorrhaging on the left brain of the larger twin. Another scan on the fifteenth day showed an "extension of the lesion" and more damage to the right brain. It was very serious, the parents were told. Their baby would most certainly develop spasticity in both arms and legs, her vision would be abnormal, and she would probably be mentally retarded. Her doctors were uncertain whether she would even be able to sit up. The baby was discharged from the hospital after two and a half months, and, at that time, all four limbs were moving normally and she was gaining weight and eating normally. The long-term prognosis for this child to lead a normal life was not, however, hopeful.

Hyperbaric oxygen therapy was recommended—one hour sessions at 2 ATA, six days a week for three months, five days a week for three more months, and finally, three sessions a week until the baby had fulfilled nine months of HBOT. At eighteen months, the child was alert, had some coordination, and showed no evidence of spasticity, although her twin was obviously far ahead of her in development. The report does state, however, that HBOT was recently renewed because there was some evidence of mild spasticity developing in her right leg. Her progress indicates that it is unlikely that any dramatic deterioration will take place, but her physicians are quick to point out that she may, at some point, still manifest symptoms of the damage to her brain. On the other hand, she continues to be very alert and responsive. Her head control is slowly developing, she is beginning to crawl, and she is able to put objects in her mouth.

In my terms, this is a success story, although the ending is hardly written. From a prognosis as dire as the one she received at birth, her slow-but-sure progress over eighteen months certainly gives us hope that children with cerebral palsy can benefit from HBOT and have the possibility of enjoying active lives, even without complete cures. The opportunities for this possibility, however, will come only if the hospital or institution providing treatment is equipped with hyperbaric chambers that can be used to treat this formidable condition, not to mention the other illnesses and conditions that can benefit from HBOT.

HBOT and Cerebral Palsy

Rebecca Serpellini was diagnosed at ten months old with cerebral palsy. I now believe that had she been treated with hyperbaric oxygen therapy when she first exhibited signs of brain damage shortly after her birth, she would be normal today.

Rebecca's mom, Yvette, told me how she came to find out about HBOT. They live in Ontario, Canada, and were watching the news one night when a story caught her attention. It was about a Montreal woman whose four-year-old twin boys were born prematurely and were subsequently diagnosed with cerebral palsy, just like Rebecca. But the twins' mother was talking about how she immediately took her boys to the United Kingdom for a treatment called hyperbaric oxygen therapy. She said that after only two weeks of treatment, their condition was very much improved. And the neurologist who is the twins' physician reported the astonishing results of the treatments. One of the boys no longer needed his leg braces and was totally functional. The other twin was now sitting up alone and feeding himself, and his spasticity (the stiffness in his muscles) had decreased by 60 to 70 percent. The videos shot before and after the treatments verified how greatly the boys' conditions had improved.

After seeing the remarkable improvement of these twins, McGill University in Montreal carried out a pilot project in 1999, using HBOT to treat twenty-five children with cerebral palsy. Its promising results convinced the Canadian government to authorize a $1.2 million grant to further study the effects of HBOT on cerebral palsy.

Meantime, spurred on by the initial television report on the twins, Mrs. Serpellini began lobbying the Ontario government to provide funding for this controversial treatment. The media covered her initiative and the response from the public was immediate. The Serpellinis, along with other parents of children with cerebral palsy, decided to create a foundation to treat affected children with hyperbaric medicine so others would not have to live with the debilitating disease, as their children did. And they are not alone. Determined parents from all over North America are following their example, even though their effort to raise the consciousness of the medical establishment is making slow progress. However, the spark has already been ignited to put more light on this remarkable treatment—their children's lifesaver.

Two Brothers with Autism

I have been treating two brothers diagnosed with autism. The younger one, two-and-a-half-year-old Jonathan, was the product of a normal delivery by his thirty-five-year-old mother. Because he had severe food allergies, eczema, and hyperactivity, Jonathan had previously been treated for the allergies by homeopathic physicians, so his family was familiar with complementary medicine. When I first saw him, his verbal development was very poor—he had a vocabulary of less than ten words.

I started him on hyperbaric oxygen therapy for five sessions at 1.5 ATA, increasing the rest of the sessions to 1.75 ATA. He has currently had forty-seven treatments. When he began HBOT, he made almost no sounds, but remarkably, after only the sixteenth treatment, he began babbling. His mother was very excited to see such dramatic improvement so quickly. She could hardly believe it. After his forty-seventh HBOT session, the therapist reported that when she said "Hi!" to Jonathan, he said "Hi!" back, making eye contact with her and even smiling. This may seem to be a small achievement, but to parents of autistic children, it is a major sign of improvement. Lack of eye contact and emotional expression are typical symptoms of autism, and although these children sometimes make eye contact with a parent, or maybe even both parents, the improvement does not often include people outside the family.

Jonathan's older brother, Alex, is also autistic and came to me with the same symptoms of food allergies, eczema, and hyperactivity. Like his younger brother, Alex had a normal birth, but had not yet spoken a single word. After more than eighty sessions of HBOT, starting at 1.5 ATA and increasing to 1.75 ATA, he is now speaking in full sentences that make sense. His treatments have been completed, but he still accompanies his brother to visit our center and answers any questions we ask him. The staff reports he seems to act like any normal four year old although he continues to be hyperactive. His father reported that after the first few sessions, he had noticed a lessening of the hyperactivity, but since then there has been no observable change in that behavior. Although many autistic children are hyperactive, it is not particularly considered a symptom of autism. I asked the technician how she would rank his progress on a scale of 0–10—with 0 being no improvement, and 10 being cured. She rated him a 6. For a child with autism, a 60-percent improvement in what appeared to be an intractable case is remarkable.

AUTISM

Autism is a neurological disorder that affects young children. It is treated symptomatically since we do not yet know very much about why it develops. Autism shows up as developmental problems—an inability to socialize, a lack of language and comprehension skills, retarded physical development, and even aggressive, uncontrollable behavior. One in 500 children is autistic, and boys are four times as likely as girls to be affected. The symptoms are evident by the time a child is three years old, but children vary widely from being mildly to seriously impaired.

Educational/behavioral therapies that focus on the individual child's need for structured skill training are the most frequently applied treatments. Experienced therapists can work intensively with impaired children and can very often achieve improvements in all areas, particularly with social skills and language. Drug therapies are commonly used to control behaviors that are physically harmful to these children and those around them. The purpose of giving these medications to autistic children is to affect the levels of serotonin in their brains—serotonin is the chemical that controls mood and mental activity. But most specialists are reluctant to use drugs unless other therapies prove ineffective.

There is no known cure for autism, primarily because there is no known cause for the disorder. I believe, however, that the use of hyperbaric oxygen therapy for autism is a direction that needs further exploration; in a very small study,[7] HBOT has already shown that it can improve the symptoms of autism in a relatively short time. Three children who had demonstrated highly aggressive behavior—they flew into rages and tantrums, were unable to communicate with others, exhibited no ability to make direct eye contact, and could not understand verbal commands—made marked progress after HBOT treatments, which pre- and post-SPECT brain scans confirmed. The children were treated for eight weeks, an hour a day for five consecutive days, with two days off each week. The forty treatments were conducted at 1.5 ATA to 1.75 ATA.

These may be very small samples, but in the treatment of the conditions and diseases that currently trouble the people I see, conventional approaches work in some cases and not in others. HBOT, on the other hand, was very successful in treating *all* these autistic children. And in one of the cases cited, the SPECT scan provided definitive proof of enhanced brain function. Does this mean we have found the cure for autism?

We simply don't know because the studies are not yet large enough to give us any definitive answers. But, if an autistic child is not responding to conventional treatments, I believe parents should consider HBOT as a serious option, particularly since there have been few, if any, side effects reported with the treatment.

PART TWO

Hydrogen Peroxide Therapy and Ozone Therapy

Hydrogen Peroxide

*I*consider the use of hydrogen peroxide one of the most important treatments in my medical kit bag. It is an oxygen therapy, and when used under medically approved conditions, it works very effectively alone or in combination with other methods to enhance the immune system and bring ailing people back to health. The hydrogen peroxide compound I use is created in the laboratory, but it is important to know that hydrogen peroxide is also produced naturally in our own bodies. Its purpose is to help the immune system function properly. The granulocytes, a class of white blood cells that fight infection, produce hydrogen peroxide. This compound is also important in the process of breaking down carbohydrates, fats, protein, minerals, and vitamins in order to release the body's energy. It helps to regulate hormones and is necessary in the production of estrogen, progesterone, and thyroxin. When the body is attacked by viruses, bacteria, various fungi, or parasites, the immune system goes into action, which often depletes the body's ability to produce hydrogen peroxide and, consequently, robs the cells of needed oxygen.

Hydrogen peroxide occurs naturally in nature as well, along with ozone, more fully discussed in Chapter 7. Ozone and hydrogen peroxide are very closely related. Hydrogen peroxide is made up of two hydrogen atoms and two oxygen atoms (H_2O_2), and is created in the atmosphere when ultraviolet light meets the element oxygen in the presence of moisture. Pure oxygen in science is designated as (O), but when it is free floating in the environment, it is designated as (O_2). And when you add an extra atom of oxygen (O_3) it is called ozone. When ozone (O_3) comes in contact with water (H_2O)—two atoms of hydrogen, one of oxygen—the extra atom splits off and combines with the water to become H_2O_2 or hydrogen peroxide. In a therapeutic sense, the lab versions of both are able to destroy bacteria, viruses, and even tumors. They have very strong anecdotal support, as well as positive results from validated research studies.

Hydrogen peroxide and ozone are known to be effective treatments as oxygenators—compounds that help increase oxygen to body systems. They are also oxidators—compounds that facilitate oxidation, an essential body process by which oxygen combines with another substance. But given a choice, in my practice I prefer hydrogen peroxide therapy to ozone therapy for its ease of oxygen delivery to the cellular level in the body.

In the early part of the nineteenth century, Dr. Louis-Jacques Thenard, a French chemist, was reputedly the first person to discover hydrogen peroxide, calling it "l'eau oxygène," or oxygenated water. But hydrogen peroxide had, in fact, been used in medicine in America almost simultaneously with its European discovery. Dr. I. N. Love, a St. Louis physician, first reported his findings in a paper given at the St. Louis Medical Society. He had treated his patients with hydrogen peroxide—diluting it with water and administering it with a syringe through the nostrils—for a number of diseases, including diphtheria, hay fever, scarlet fever, tonsillitis, and whooping cough. It was reported that all of them had experienced improvement in their conditions, so it is clear that during this time the exploration of medical uses for H_2O_2 was expanding. Commercial uses for hydrogen peroxide as a disinfectant, oxidizing agent, and non-polluting bleaching agent had already been developed in the mid-1800s, but no reports of medical uses for this useful substance turn up in the medical literature until about 1916 when *The Lancet*—the noted British medical journal—discussed H_2O_2 therapy for the first time. The English physicians F. W. Turnicliffe and G. F. Stebbing are believed to be the first medical doctors to produce therapeutic results by delivering H_2O_2 to human beings intravenously.

Not long after, in 1920, *The Lancet* reported that British physicians T. H. Oliver and B. C. Cantab used hydrogen peroxide to treat pneumonia cases in India. At the time, Indian troops were experiencing an 80 percent mortality rate from the disease. Despite warnings that injecting H_2O_2 might cause gas embolism (strokes resulting from bubbles in the brain), soldiers considered hopeless were treated, and 50 percent of them—thirteen out of twenty-five cases—survived! In 1940, Dr. Inderjit Singh, one of the pioneer researchers in hydrogen peroxide therapy, found that intravenous oxygen could keep dogs alive for sixteen minutes without "any air going through the lungs." Before using H_2O_2, the animals might have survived only three or four minutes.

In the next twenty years, physicians around the world who believed strongly in the therapeutic value of H_2O_2 conducted a number of research studies, as for example, the Baylor University Medical Center research into the therapeutic use of H_2O_2 in both animals and humans in the 1960s. The fact that oxygen could be delivered into living tissue through an injection of H_2O_2 reinforced what was known about H_2O_2 twenty years earlier—that hydrogen peroxide was therapeutically viable and could be delivered to a patient simply and inexpensively.

The story of hydrogen peroxide therapy and its slow progress toward recognition parallels the story of other approaches that were once considered mainstream before being replaced by a new treatment concept (drugs) that had physician approval, commercial backing, and promotional support—a necessity for the launch of any new treatment.

The high visibility of drug therapies, which began just as H_2O_2 was on its way to establishing credibility, was made possible by the pharmaceutical companies, particularly in the United States. These well-financed corporations quickly realized that drugs could be sold commercially in retail stores. Even prestigious journals such as *The Journal of the American Medical Association* (*JAMA*) were eager to report the findings of research conducted with pharmaceutical industry funding. Today, the strong connection between the pharmaceutical industry and physicians has been firmly established, but the public has not been aware of how interconnected that relationship has been. Recently, *The New York Times* reported that "a survey of medical experts who write guidelines for treating conditions like heart disease, depression, and diabetes, has found that nearly nine out of ten have financial ties to the pharmaceutical industry, and the ties are almost never disclosed." Financial conflicts of interest are, of course, the main issue for *The New York Times*. What concerns me the most, however, is that treatments that are not drug-based find it impossible to get funding for research. In the United States, solid and expensive research must have pharmaceutical industry support in order to be conducted in the first place, and then to be promoted to a larger public after the results are known.

So, back then as now, with even as persuasive a case as proponents of hydrogen peroxide therapy (along with herbal approaches, homeopathy, hyperbaric oxygen therapy, and others) could make, the research dollars were hard to come by. Drug treatments, it seemed, were the only therapeutic approaches offered, and the news of their successes was so widely promoted that it made any other approach appear less effective and certainly less up to date. The ease of delivery and the effectiveness of the treatments were popular with both the physicians and the public. It didn't take long before the use of drug treatments almost eliminated the availability of any other previously sanctioned treatments. It was, of course, shortsighted because it overlooked what drugs could *not* do.

Enamored of drug therapy, the doctors and the public alike would take another thirty-five years to realize that hydrogen peroxide therapy and hyperbaric oxygen therapy had been effective treatments and should again be taken seriously. And physicians only began returning to medical concepts that had been effective before the advent of drugs because they became concerned by the side effects of most drugs. They also realized that diseases such as cancer and heart disease were occurring in almost epidemic proportions, despite almost miraculous developments in surgical techniques. In the process of their rediscovery, they found that in the United States and other countries, there had been ongoing research studies, particularly on hydrogen peroxide therapy and hyperbaric oxygen therapy, and that the evidence showing the effectiveness of these therapies had slowly been mounting.

Most people know hydrogen peroxide as the colorless liquid kept in the bathroom to be used as a mouthwash or as a disinfectant or antiseptic to treat minor scratches or wounds. This form of hydrogen peroxide is called 3 percent grade, and should not be taken into the body. It also comes in higher grades. Six percent is used to bleach hair. Thirty percent hydrogen peroxide is the highly concentrated version used in medical research. It is toxic and should not be ingested either, but this is the grade of hydrogen peroxide that, mixed with water, we use therapeutically. Thirty-five percent food grade is commonly used as a disinfectant by the food and dairy industries. It is nontoxic and, when mixed with water, can keep fresh foods free of bacteria. Ninety-percent grade hydrogen peroxide is highly combustible, an unstable compound used mostly by the military, never medically.

As discussed in the Introduction, one of the medical community's criticisms of hydrogen peroxide is on the chemical level because they think it is possible that hydrogen peroxide, as medical treatment, can lead to an uncontrolled production of free radicals. Instead of enhancing the healing process, the argument goes, it can cause cell damage in the body. Free-radical formation, as we said, refers to molecules that have an unpaired electron—stable molecules have paired electrons. In nature, the free-radical electron, wanting stability, steals an electron from a stable molecule, thereby destabilizing it. That molecule—now minus an electron—becomes a free radical itself and looks around to connect with a balancing electron. The process continues, setting in motion a chain reaction that affects other molecules. You can see that, within the body, one free-radical electron can quickly cause structural damage in other molecules, and with an excess of free radicals, cell damage to the body can be a very serious possibility.

On the other hand, free radicals such as hydroxyl, among others formed from hydrogen peroxide, have important properties essential to a well-functioning system. They produce energy in the body. They kill bacteria and viruses. They can regulate hormones. These are essential qualities in treating disease and bringing our bodies back to health. Conventional medicine is concerned that using hydrogen peroxide as a therapy "can lead to uncontrolled production of free radicals," and links this chain reaction of free radicals to various degenerative diseases, such as arthritis, cancer, and diabetes. The issue in using hydrogen peroxide is, therefore, how to gain the benefit of free radicals while limiting their potential for reproducing out of control.

After many years of prescribing hydrogen peroxide therapy to my patients, I know it is possible to harness only the positive aspects of free-radical production. Also, by using hydrogen peroxide responsibly, it is possible to bring oxygen directly to the cell level by actually killing disease agents. I have found that using small amounts of the compound can strengthen the immune system. One of the properties of hydrogen peroxide is to make T cells stronger, consequently more resistant to oxidation and more likely to develop healthy new cells.

The late Dr. Charles Farr, Founder and Medical Director of the International Oxidative Medicine Association, and a nominee for the Nobel Prize in Medicine in 1993, is quoted in Nathaniel Altman's excellent book *Oxygen Healing Therapies,* saying that he believes strongly in the thera-

Samantha's Litany of Problems

"I'm tired of being sick," Samantha said, slumped in her chair in my office. Patients often arrive at my office with some version of the same generalized complaint. They feel terrible and they despair because there are so many things wrong with them. Samantha's litany of physical problems was overwhelming—abdominal pain, bloating, chronic viral attacks, headaches, lumps in her breast (due to fibrocystic breasts), and vaginal dryness, as well as anxiety attacks and night sweats that constantly disturbed her sleep. In addition, she had chronic fatigue syndrome, irritable bowel syndrome, and hypometabolism (a sluggish thyroid system), although the blood work for her thyroid function was perfectly normal. She was also troubled by candidiasis and a chronic urinary tract infection. All this, and a life-numbing depression.

Thirty-nine years old and from Chile, Samantha only came to see me at her brother's insistence—he was my patient, too. Her depression began as a teenager, she said, and she had tried to commit suicide twice. In 1998, she had a hysterectomy for endometriosis and was given Premarin, an estrogen product made from mare's urine, but had stopped taking it ten months before she came to see me. Some of her problems came from the fact that she had not been on any hormone replacement for almost a year. I recommended a natural estrogen and progesterone to relieve the menopausal symptoms—mood swings, night sweats, and vaginal dryness.

peutic potential of hydrogen peroxide. His discovery that "hydrogen peroxide leads to the formation of hydroxyl radicals *only* under special circumstances, primarily when ferrous oxide is present,"[1] is an important one. It offers a set of methods to physicians who may want to use this treatment, but are concerned about the issue of free radicals. (In excessive amounts, hydroxyl free radicals in the body have been linked to the destruction of cell membranes and to genetic mutations.) Dr. Farr found that hydrogen peroxide *without* the presence of iron (no iron supplements should be taken when this therapy is used) converts to oxygen by means of the enzyme catalase, which, in turn, makes hydrogen peroxide a benefit to the body. He says, "One molecule of catalase can convert millions of molecules of hydrogen peroxide into oxygen and water within seconds, and is the body's first line of defense against hydroxyl radical formation."

We needed to deal with Samantha's allergic reaction to candida immediately because it was depressing her immune system. Candida, which is normally present in the body, is a potentially lethal kind of yeast. When stimulated by antibiotics, birth control pills, estrogen, and a poor diet consisting of too much sugar and carbohydrates, yeast can be overproduced in the body, releasing toxins. Yeast also has the potential to produce antigens—foreign substances—that can overwhelm the antibodies protecting the body. That is what had happened in Samantha's case. She had developed multiple allergies. I started her on allergy injections and put her on my anti-yeast FAVER diet—Fish, All meats, Vegetables, Eggs, and Rice cakes.[2]

I then recommended injections of pure pharmaceutical grade hydrogen peroxide three times a week for two months. I knew that once we dealt with the allergies, we needed to stimulate her immune system and bring oxygen directly to her cells so we could revitalize a seriously weakened body.

When Samantha came to see me four and a half months later, she had lost nineteen pounds and most of her symptoms were gone. She was still feeling a little tired but said she was 40 percent better and getting stronger. The hydrogen peroxide infusions made her feel much better, because it was stimulating her own antioxidant potential and enhancing her body's ability to use the oxygen in her body efficiently. I recommended that she continue the treatment once a week until her energy came back and she could finally say she felt well. She did, and now she feels like a new person.

This discovery should allay some of the medical community's negative attitude toward the use of hydrogen peroxide and allow it to focus instead on the many benefits that can accrue with this therapy.

I believe that one very effective way to counteract the buildup of free radicals is to make sure that patients are also on a health program that features a regular intake of antioxidants through nutritional supplements and a diet that includes plenty of fresh fruits and vegetables.

We cannot underestimate Dr. Farr's contribution to the wealth of knowledge on hydrogen peroxide. (See Chapter 1.) His work is responsible for our ability to use oxygen therapeutically today. His professional degrees were in both medicine and pharmacology, and he understood the importance of research, and of applying his discoveries to the treatment of patients, once he saw that H_2O_2, used appropriately, was a compound that produced few, if any, side effects. Dr. Farr is credited with pioneering the successful treatment of many diseases using intravenous injections of hydrogen peroxide dilutions. No one has conducted more clinical studies on H_2O_2 therapy and chelation therapy than Dr. Farr, but for most of his life, his remarkable work was unrecognized by the medical profession in the United States. Outside America, however, researchers and medical professionals had watched the progress of his work closely, and his nomination for the Nobel Prize in Medicine for his work on hydrogen peroxide brought much-needed attention to all the research on biological oxidation. Allergies, asthma, autoimmune diseases (rheumatoid arthritis and lupus), bronchitis, chronic fatigue syndrome, heart disease, influenza, shingles, and many other chronic conditions and diseases plaguing people today have all been treated with H_2O_2, with positive results ranging from improvement to cure.

However, it continues to be an uphill struggle to make his work visible to a broader public in the United States, physicians included. Since 1920, there have been more than 6,000 scientific articles published on hydrogen peroxide as a therapeutic process. In my opinion, it is certainly time for this important therapeutic approach to receive broader acceptance and use to benefit the many ill patients for whom drugs have not brought relief from illness—and certainly no cure.

Understanding the actual physiological effects of hydrogen peroxide on the body highlights the value of H_2O_2 as a therapeutic compound. Hydrogen peroxide has a definite metabolic effect on the body—in other words, it encourages the chemical and physical processes in the body and helps release energy, specifically by combining with iodine to maintain a healthy functioning thyroid gland. It also is important to the production of progesterone—an essential hormone that aids in reproduction. Another of its jobs is prostaglandin synthesis, helping to control the powerful hormones and hormonelike substances that are involved in maintaining vital body processes. H_2O_2 also helps to stimulate dopamine, a neurotransmitter that is necessary for proper nerve function in the brain. It mimics the hormone insulin in the body, as well; insulin is essential in the treatment of diabetes.

H_2O_2 can aid the vessels that carry blood and lymph throughout the body. It both supports vasodilation, the widening of cerebral and coronary arteries and peripheral vessels, and helps prevent vasoconstriction, the narrowing of blood vessels. H_2O_2 also has the capacity to help increase oxygenation in pulmonary or lung tissue.

Hydrogen peroxide is particularly useful in encouraging the immune system to function effectively. First of all, it stimulates the production of lymphocytes (white blood cells), known as T-helper cells, which help to improve the integrity of the immune system. H_2O_2 also stimulates gamma interferon, a protein that inhibits the growth of viruses and decreases the activity of B cells, special types of lymphocytes that produce antibodies. It can also regulate the immune system, as well as help to manage an inflammatory response in the body—when tissues or organs become inflamed in response to infection.

There are many other functions of hydrogen peroxide discussed in medical books and journals that are well understood by many physicians. That is why I prescribe it for my patients who can benefit from it, without hesitation.

Clinical Uses of Hydrogen Peroxide

W hether it is talking to patients or convincing the medical community at large, one of the most difficult problems for me is overcoming the skepticism regarding the use of hydrogen peroxide as a therapeutic treatment. People tend to associate it only with its commercial use. This is because for generations, hydrogen peroxide's major uses have been in industry, primarily in the chemical, mining, and textile fields, although it has also been used successfully in agriculture and for rocket fuel.

Used medically since 1888, it is one of those therapies that, despite its success, tends to be regarded suspiciously. Perhaps its easy accessibility and the fact that it is an inexpensive, natural substance tends to hamper its wider acceptance as a credible medical treatment. Also, hydrogen peroxide is known as a home remedy, anecdotally reported to relieve stiff joints, rashes, and fungal infections, which tends to relegate it to first-aid status rather than enhance its use as an effective treatment for serious illnesses.

Further, too many of the articles and books written on the subject of hydrogen peroxide are diminished by their desire to promote its use—mostly from a sincere belief in the treatment—and they end up leaving readers with the distinct impression that it is a cure-all. On the Internet and in other media, the list of uses for hydrogen peroxide range from treating the flu to Parkinson's disease—with Alzheimer's disease, irregular heartbeats, and rheumatoid arthritis in between. Theoretically and practically, this is actually true. Researchers and scientists confirm that, because hydrogen peroxide can kill some very mean pathogens and even some tumor cells, it has been used in the treatment of more than thirty diseases with "varying degrees of success."[1] But that wide a range of treatments makes most people suspicious of its effectiveness, and they would rather "throw the baby out with the bathwater" than explore the real possibility of improved health. The problem in the twenty-first century is that we want definitive *cures* for the prevalent diseases of our time. In some instances, hydrogen peroxide may provide a cure; in others, the disease state is improved. Because this substance has such remarkable qualities when applied to the human body, a healthier state is not only possible, but also probable. Having said that, I also believe that using hydrogen peroxide alone in the treatment of most diseases and conditions may not be sufficient to bring a person back to full health. It often takes medical detective work to diagnose an illness and a combination of treatments to take care of all the complaints and symptoms. Unfortunately, illnesses, particularly chronic conditions, aren't often cured with a single method. But I have found that hydrogen peroxide is one of the most effective, and because it has few, if any, side effects, I often prescribe its use as an initial treatment. Whether conventional or alternative treatment is called for, someone has to be in charge of the patient's care, first acting as a medical detective, then going on to discover the best combinations of treatments for the condition. Doing it on your own is frustrating and, in my experience, doesn't work most of the time except when you treat normal illness, such as minor colds, cuts, bruises, or general fatigue. Will it harm you to treat yourself with hydrogen peroxide therapy? No, not as long as you refrain from ingesting it. The 3 percent hydrogen peroxide, the most widely available strength, can safely be used on the body as a disinfectant, or in the kitchen and bathroom for general cleaning.

Here's the truth about the hydrogen peroxide I use. The 30 percent reagent grade developed for medical purposes *does* have very broad use and minimal, if any, side effects. But the treatment with this grade *must* be monitored by a physician who is experienced in the use of this therapy. It is not a self-help treatment. The uses for hydrogen peroxide that are suggested in books on home remedies or folk medicine may or may not have some effect when used for treatment of minor health conditions. But when it comes to treating serious illness and chronic conditions, it is essential to be under the watchful care of a qualified medical professional. Since each of us has a different physical makeup and different medical histories,

Linda's Miraculous Recovery

Linda, a forty-three-year-old practicing psychotherapist, heard me discussing my approach to medicine on my radio program, and had an intuitive feeling that I might be able to help her. Perhaps she responded to my conviction that practicing medicine is detective work. Finding out why someone is ill is often a matter of experienced trial and error, but when a treatment works, we know because the person's condition improves. And if we seriously explore the possibilities, I know that there will eventually be an answer and a solution in most cases.

Linda had seen many other physicians before coming to me with her unique complaint. She was experiencing pain along the right side of her body, from her head down to her toes. It was as if her body was split down the middle. No pain at all on the left side. Beyond that, her memory had degenerated. She had no appetite, and she was depressed, nauseous, and tired, but couldn't sleep.

When Linda came to me, she was convinced she had Lyme disease because a prior test had shown she was mildly positive, although a subsequent one came back negative, according to her doctor at the time. After listening to her, I thought she might have chronic fatigue immune dysfunction syndrome, and because she was having irregular periods, I also thought she might be in perimenopause. But to remove all her doubts, I decided to have her tested again for Lyme disease. While we waited for results, we began a month-long treatment with the antibiotics Flagyl and Augmentin—common for Lyme disease—just in case she did have it. At the same time, I recommended twenty sessions of hyperbaric oxygen therapy with 2.4 atmosphere absolute ATA—the HBOT protocol for Lyme disease. After the treatment was completed, her symptoms seemed to be taken care of, but she experienced two nights of diarrhea afterward, and then the pain on the right side of her body returned. Needless to say, we were both disappointed. The blood work came back negative for Lyme disease so we could now rule that out once and for all.

Next, we tried intravenous hydrogen peroxide three times a week, along with five or six treatments of HBOT, acupuncture, and supplementation with vitamins, minerals, amino acids, and fatty acids. When she came to see me after six weeks, Linda was feeling 30 to 40 percent better, so I knew we were on the right track. But she still had the same level of pain on the right side of her face. Maybe she had fibromyalgia on the right side, along with chronic fatigue, which affects muscles and glands and is extremely painful. Another possibility was allergies. We did allergy tests and discovered she was allergic to almost everything—food, including beef, eggplant, and milk; dust; feathers; mold; and tobacco.

For two more months we continued with intravenous hydrogen peroxide, allergy injections, and acupuncture, and we added chelation therapy, a process by which heavy metals are captured by EDTA, a synthetic amino acid, and taken out of the body through the kidneys. This chelating process seems to turn on the body's repair mechanisms, leading to a softening of abnormally hardened blood vessel walls. It removes atherosclerotic plaque, the fatty "rust" that blocks arteries and leads to heart attacks, strokes, or gangrene.

Two months later, Linda returned. She said she had never felt better. We had definitely established that the allergies, in combination with chronic fatigue and fibromyalgia, were the causes of her strange condition. The treatment consisted of hydrogen peroxide therapy, hyperbaric oxygen therapy, acupuncture, change of diet, the addition of nutrients, and finally, chelation therapy. And it worked. The last time I saw her, she asked me for health certification papers for her employer. It took four and a half months of treatment, but the mystery was finally solved.

In Linda's case, intravenous hydrogen peroxide therapy was just one of the many complementary treatments used to finally deliver a cure. That is why I object to creating any mistaken perception that a single mode of treatment always works to cure a disease or condition. Linda's health improved primarily because both hydrogen peroxide therapy and hyperbaric oxygen therapy were infusing her body with maximum amounts of oxygen to trigger her immune system and allowing it to work better and make her stronger. The chelation cleansed her body of heavy metals and the right foods and supplements refueled her body, which was also stimulated by the acupuncture to rebalance her energy, her flow of *qi*. Together, it was a forceful treatment program designed specifically and individually for Linda. Each person's body is unique, and what works for one person probably won't work for someone else. As a doctor, I can use many tools for healing, and will pass by a procedure only when it is proven to be ineffective, either on its own or in combination with some other approach.

there are many variables, including dosage, length, and frequency of treatment, that demand the experience of a knowledgeable practitioner.

The reason hydrogen peroxide is included in this book on oxygen therapies and the reason I use it in my practice is because hydrogen peroxide has a remarkable quality as an oxygenator, delivering the healing element of oxygen to the blood, stimulating oxidative enzymes, and in general, increasing the body's capacity to use the oxygen it has.

As a complementary physician, I use oxygen as a treatment whenever possible, and I use the best possible delivery system I can. It is one of the few elements I know that can kill pathogens, naturally heal the body, encourage the immune system to function, and stimulate the body's processes to revitalize.

HOW HYDROGEN PEROXIDE IS ADMINISTERED

In my practice, I only use intravenous injections. At the CAM Institute for Integrative Therapies—a complementary medical facility in Brooklyn, New York, where I am the medical director, we dilute 3 cc of 3 percent reagent-grade hydrogen peroxide with 250 cc NACl (sodium chloride) solution and infuse it intravenously into a patient, for forty-five minutes to an hour. Three infusions a week for up to three or four months is not unusual, and sometimes a follow-up once a week is necessary. The injections cost $100 per infusion and, unfortunately, are not covered by insurance unless a patient has a flexible benefit package. Some companies will allow employees to put aside a certain amount of money in a special fund set up by an insurance company—usually $1,000—deducted from a paycheck in equal amounts over twelve months. The money must be used for medical treatments by acupuncturists, chiropractors, dentists, doctors, and so on, or used to pay for medically related purchases, such as glasses or crutches—all of which are expenses that are not included in normal insurance plans. The employee is required to pay for the treatment or purchase out of pocket, then submit the receipt to the insurer to get reimbursed for the expense. If the entire amount is not spent within the year, the employee loses the balance to the insurance company, which also makes its money on the interest. If you know you will be having such medical expenses during the year, it is a good way to have at least $1,000 of the total reimbursed. Contact your health benefits coordinator at your workplace, or call your insurance company for more information about *Flexible Benefits*.

Matthew's Complicated Case History

When Matthew came to me, he claimed to know all about alternative and conventional medicine. He had tried everything and nothing seemed to work. As an expert on his own condition, Matthew was the nightmare patient for any physician because he thought he knew it all. He came to me with a treatment plan he had worked out on his own, and he wanted me to follow it.

Matthew complained of extreme fatigue that was so severe he could work only four hours at a time. He also had orthostatic hypertension, blood pressure that rises when standing up. He said he'd had a low body temperature for about five years and that he was dizzy, had perpetually cold feet and hands, and had painful arthritis. At one point, his arthritis was treated with nonsteroidal anti-inflammatory drugs (NSAIDs). He had a history of alcohol abuse but had stopped drinking about a year and a half before coming to see me. Several alternative physicians had diagnosed him with "yeast and parasite" problems. Nystatin had been prescribed for candidiasis, but he had refused to take it. Matthew was the kind of patient who could drive even a patient doctor to impatience. In his case, however, my medical interest far outweighed my frustration.

I suspected that, in addition to hypometabolism/hypothyroidism—a sluggish function of the thyroid gland—he probably had heavy metal toxicity. His

As I said, other applications of hydrogen peroxide are often suggested and although you cannot argue with the success that is reported, I personally have seldom seen consistent results when hydrogen peroxide is used for bathing or taken orally.

MEDICAL INDICATIONS FOR TREATMENT WITH HYDROGEN PEROXIDE

It is important for anyone who has been diagnosed with medical problems and has received treatment from conventional physicians, or is on regular medications, to be aware of H_2O_2 as an option. In most cases, the treatment can be administered along with conventional care.

Many patients with the conditions, diseases, or problems numbered below have seen improvement after a course of treatment with hydrogen peroxide. Some have even been cured. But, in my opinion, simply knowing there are viable options for sick people who want to feel better, options urine test confirmed my diagnosis. As it turned out, Matthew had had a mercury toxicity in the past. He also tested positive for Epstein-Barr virus (EBV). For his insomnia, we recommended a workup to prepare him for a sleep study.

To make sure we took care of the mercury toxicity, our first step was to start Matthew on chelation therapy, alternating it with hydrogen peroxide therapy and intravenous vitamin and mineral drips. In his adamant desire to control his treatment, Matthew continued to see other alternative practitioners and conventional doctors, but as time went on, he began to realize that the chelation and hydrogen peroxide therapies, along with our program of nutritional supplements, made him feel better. So, as we recommended, he came more often for treatment, and he has now, according to his own grudging assessment, improved 50, maybe even 60, percent.

Because Matthew had tried everything and had lost hope of ever feeling better, this approach was a miracle for him. For me, Matthew was the success of my medical life. The frustration of seeing him jump from treatment to treatment, certain that he knew what would work for him, made treating him extremely difficult. It is a good thing I am a patient physician, and his example continues to give me confidence that the frustrating work of discovering ways to combine treatments to make people feel better is worth it.

they have not yet explored, is in itself encouraging. Of course, it is always possible that an individual may not be a candidate for H_2O_2 therapy, but it is important to at least explore the possibility.

1. People experiencing cardiovascular problems, such as angina or heart attacks (coronary artery disease), could benefit from this therapy. Those who have strokes (cerebrovascular accidents), peripheral vascular conditions, or arrhythmias have seen vast improvement in their conditions.

2. Many people who have been troubled by pulmonary (lung) disease (bronchial asthma, chronic obstructive pulmonary disease, or emphysema) have, for many years, found their breathing easier and had their energy restored by a course of H_2O_2 treatments.

3. Inflammatory diseases, such as temporal arteritis or rheumatoid arthri-

tis, respond favorably to hydrogen peroxide therapy, and patients note less swelling and more movement after treatments.

Treating Maureen's Physical and Emotional Ills

Maureen had been ill with bronchial asthma for six years before she came to see me, and she has now been my patient for more than four years. She is fifty years old and has never been admitted to a hospital; she has only seen an allergist who gave her allergy injections and prescribed inhalers as treatment. Claritin was her prescription of record.

Aside from her allergies, she was emotionally stressed because her stepson had a drinking problem and her husband was unavailable. She complained, too, of having dry and itchy skin, frequent mood swings, hives, mouth sores, poor short-term memory, and a history of severe vaginal yeast problems. She had been troubled for seventeen years by irritable bowel syndrome, which was now much worse. She also had candidiasis.

I put Maureen on my anti-yeast FAVER diet, consisting of Fish, All meats (antibiotic-free), Vegetables, Eggs, and Rice cakes, to begin to deal with the candidiasis. The key to the diet is keeping the person away from yeast-containing foods, or anything that provides direct stimulation of yeast growth. She was eventually able to add limited amounts of fruits, such as apples, berries, and pears, to her diet. The diet is designed so that, as health improves, some yeast-containing or higher carbohydrate foods are added. But for patients with candidiasis, foods high in yeast, pickled or smoked foods, or foods high in sugar are off-limits.

Maureen was near menopause and also showed symptoms of a hormonal imbalance. Her estrogen, progesterone, and testosterone levels were all at the lower limits, so we prescribed natural estrogen, progesterone, and testosterone.

But it was the intravenous hydrogen peroxide three times a week for twenty weeks that began to turn around the asthma that had troubled her for so long. After these injections, she was 80 percent improved. "My energy is back," she said. Her lifetime asthma symptoms were diminished. No more congestion. Her memory returned, and her irritable bowel symptoms improved. By four months, Maureen's life was finally getting on track and was no longer consumed by illness. Now she comes in once or twice a month for maintenance hydrogen peroxide treatments.

4. People with endocrine problems have responded well to H_2O_2. The endocrine glands, like the adrenals, the pituitary, and the thyroid glands, produce one or more internal secretions (hormones) that are introduced directly into the bloodstream and carried to the parts of the body they regulate. Type II diabetes and hypothyroidism are just some of the conditions related to hormone regulation that have been improved with this treatment.

5. People with neuromuscular problems, highly prevalent today and with few, if any, solutions for their various physical manifestations, respond very well to hydrogen peroxide. Such conditions as cluster, migraine, or vascular headaches can be cured. Chronic pain syndrome can see great improvement, and even very serious neuromuscular conditions, such as multiple sclerosis or Parkinson's disease, can be improved, although real cures are seldom reported. People treated with H_2O_2 therapy do find, however, that the therapy gives them more control over their limbs and bodies and they feel stronger. Alzheimer's disease–related dementia, different from vascular dementia, does not respond to HBOT, but it does respond favorably to a course of treatment with hydrogen peroxide.

6. Infectious diseases are very good candidates for treatment with H_2O_2. Chronic bacterial infection, fungi (*Aspergillus fumigatus, Blastomyces,* or *Candida species*), parasites (*Entamoeba histolytica, Pneumocytsis carinii,* or *Trichomonas vaginalis*), viruses (herpes virus, CMV, HIV, and others) are all very effectively treated with hydrogen peroxide.

The patients I have discussed in my case histories are typical of the people I see daily. They moved from a state of being sick to a state of being well. It is no small thing these days to be able to consult with a doctor who knows your total case history and is committed to work at discovering what is wrong, why you're sick, and exploring solutions. Our patients are the source of new and continuing knowledge. Treating them, we learn not to take anything for granted and to follow up on every lead.

A complementary physician relies on referrals from patients who have received treatment that improved their health, whose personal experience with complementary medicine changed their lives. We in complementary medicine have the advantage that, as medical doctors, we not only have access to conventional diagnostic equipment, pharmaceuticals, surgery, and the privilege of consulting specialists when necessary, but we are also committed to treating the whole mind/body. This combination of access, interest, knowledge, and skill is, in my opinion, the role of medicine today. Because it works, it is necessary. With none of established medicine's bias against natural healing, we can prescribe herbs and other supplements, we understand and promote the value of food as a healing tool, and we use treatments such as hydrogen peroxide to improve health with few side effects. It is the best of all medical worlds in which to practice.

Ozone Therapy: What Do We Know?

Ozone can perform what oxygen cannot.
—ERWIN PAYR, M.D.

*I*n recent years, ozone has become a hot topic for environmentalists. It is a colorless gas constantly being formed some "twenty to thirty kilometers above the earth's surface as a result of ultraviolet radiation from the sun continuously acting on atmospheric oxygen."[1] It surrounds the planet, protecting all living things from the harmful effects of the sun's ultraviolet rays. Its importance to us cannot be underestimated. A serious result of our contemporary consumer culture is that the protective ozone has thinned—gaping holes have even been observed in some places—and we are now exposed to the direct power of the sun's ultraviolet rays, with negative consequences. The major cause of this thinning out of the ozone is the release of chlorofluorocarbons into the atmosphere from aerosol containers, refrigerators, and air conditioners. Recently, steps have been taken by manufacturers in the United States to comply with governmental regulations aimed at minimizing the release of these chlorofluorocarbons, but this is a world problem that affects the health of all human beings and the vitality of our environment. We are seeing more skin cancer. Our immune systems have been weakened and more immune-related diseases are being reported. Closer to Earth, ozone combines with carbon dioxide and nitrogen, creating deadly pollution in the air we breathe and causing any number of lung-related diseases. So, what we know about ozone is only the bad news.

But there is another side of ozone, and it is a far different story. Ozone has a substantive role to play as an effective medical therapy. The early history of ozone, much like that of hydrogen peroxide, shows that ozone's positive properties were being explored. In Germany, in 1901, ozone was used to purify water and, in 1915, to treat skin diseases. During World War I, the Germans used ozone to treat battle wounds and infections. But it was not until 1945 that Dr. Erwin Payr, a surgeon, used ozone medically by injecting it intravenously into patients with circulatory problems. Since then, more scientific and industrial uses for ozone have been developed as the technology for generating the gas has become increasingly sophisticated.

Due to its early history with ozone, Germany was one of the first countries to pioneer the use of ozone in treating a number of diseases, including cancer and HIV/AIDS. As is true with hyperbaric oxygen therapy, ozone therapy is widely known and used outside North America, but is almost unknown by physicians and health practitioners in the United States. Countries like Cuba and Russia have done research on medical ozone, and its therapeutic use has been widely documented. Both countries have socialized medicine in place, and because of this, their governments are particularly interested in developing inexpensive, effective treatments in order for their doctors to be less dependent on expensive drugs and surgical solutions for eliminating disease.

Ozone, like hydrogen peroxide, is an effective oxidizer that can kill all kinds of bacteria and viruses, including the toxins they produce. It also works quickly to destroy any number of poisonous compounds, such as chemical waste or pesticides, which makes this inexpensive substance particularly valuable as a disinfectant in purifying water.

As previously stated, ozone and hydrogen peroxide are closely related. They both destroy various pathogens and both are powerful oxygenators. They can enhance the immune system and encourage the natural production of oxygen in the body's tissues. Currently, ozone therapy is being used in many countries outside the United States to treat a broad range of conditions and ailments, including AIDS, allergies, arthritis, asthma, cancer, colitis, hepatitis, herpes, and sinusitis. Ozone is also used in dentistry. Not only is it an efficient disinfectant, but it also works to control bleeding and speed healing of sensitive tissues. Ozonated water is used by dental patients as a mouth rinse. Physicians who use ozone therapy do so simply because they see results in their patients. In America, its wider use is hampered by the reluctance of the Food and Drug Administration and the

National Institutes of Health to support clinical trials that might offer ozone therapy sufficient credibility to convince insurance carriers, physicians, and prospective patients that ozone is, first, a viable treatment and, second, an effective one.

There have recently been many controlled clinical trials that have reported results not only confirming ozone therapy as a practical treatment, but also proving that this therapy is about to make the leap from simply showing empirical evidence of effectiveness to being "scientifically founded medicine."

As reported in Dr. Renate Viebahn's book, *The Use of Ozone in Medicine,* there are six areas where treatments with ozone therapy have shown improved conditions. They are as follows:

1. **Proctology.** Two hundred forty-eight people were treated by rectal ozone/oxygen gas *insufflation* (administration of ozone through the rectum) and *"systemic efficacy"* (positive therapeutic effect on organs and system) was shown. Previously, treatment had shown improvement only in animals. Knoch, Klug, Dresden, Germany, 1992.

2. **Infectious diseases.** Thirty-two people with hepatitis B were treated in a controlled pilot study. It positively confirmed a healing rate that had already been known from a number of individual case histories. Knoch, Klug, Dresden, Germany, 1987–1988.

3. **Rheumatism/Arthritis.** Positive results of ozone treatment on 156 people with gonarthritis were reported in a study published by Riva of Bologna, Italy, 1988.

4. **Dermatology.** In a laboratory study conducted by Gehse, Gloor, Glutsch, Karlsruhe, Germany, 1990–1992, local ozone application was successfully used in combination with potassium permanganate on diseased populations of microorganisms in ulcera cruris, an ulcerous skin condition.

5. **Immunology.** Studies by Washuttl, Viebahn, Waber, Gutzen, 1992, and Bocci, 1990–1992, have demonstrated the positive effect of ozone on immunocompetent cells (cells that are able to resist infection). Of particular interest was ozone's demonstrated ability to speed up the work of interferon and interleukin 2, cellular proteins that help inhibit viral growth, as well as ozone's capacity for destroying tumors.

6. **Sports medicine.** A 1998 Viennese study conducted by Washuttl, Bachl, Jakl, Prokop, et al., demonstrated different successful methods of using ozone to treat various medical conditions resulting from sports injuries.

Physicians who practice ozone therapy have a number of methods they can use, all involving the amount of ozone added to oxygen, depending on the condition being treated and the particular medical history of the individual. The most common method is autohemotherapy. It involves taking blood with a syringe—the amount taken ranges from 10 milliliters (minor autohemotherapy) to as much as 250 milliliters (major autohemotherapy). This blood is then infused with ozone and oxygen, and in minor autohemotherapy, it gets reinjected into the person's buttock. Major autohemotherapy delivers the infused blood through an IV drip. It has been used to treat conditions such as arthritis, cancer, heart disease, and HIV. This method, first described by French researcher Lacoste in 1951, involved successful treatment of a patient threatened by amputation at the upper thigh. And, according to observations by Russian researchers Tabakova and O. Rokitansky, four out of ten people treated by ozone did not need surgery for different diseases/conditions.

Rectal insufflation is another method of ozone delivery. This procedure introduces the combination of ozone and oxygen into the body through the rectum. The substance gets absorbed by the intestines and can stay in the body anywhere from ten to twenty minutes. Other methods include water infused with ozone gas. Ozonated water is used to wash wounds and burns. It can also be used for colonics or to treat intestinal or gynecological problems. Intravenous injection of ozone is the most controversial of the methods, and those who consider it dangerous warn that there is a potential for lung clots to develop.

Delivering ozone through the skin is another method. A steam room is used, and steam, oxygen, and ozone are pumped in. The theory here is that the body absorbs the ozone through the skin. People who are convinced of the health benefits of ozone like the fact that this method is noninvasive. Ozone gas added to olive oil (ozonated oil), then applied as a salve, is also a useful form, particularly for treating fungal infections, insect bites, skin problems, or yeast infections on the skin. Cuban physicians have thoroughly researched this method of delivering ozone and have documented its effect on various physical conditions.

Other methods include autohomologous immunotherapy (AHIT), which is not approved for use in the United States. It is a complicated procedure that involves breaking down blood and urine into various cellular parts, which then undergo a number of processing steps, one of which is the addition of ozone. Depending on the individual's diagnosis, the parts are brought together, then reintroduced into the body over a period of time. Proponents of the method, mostly physicians in Europe, have found that AHIT enhances the immune system, and clinical trials show it has a positive effect on a wide range of conditions, including bronchial asthma, cancer, circulatory problems, eczema, herpes (simplex and zoster), osteo-arthritis and rheumatoid arthritis, premature aging, treatment of burns, and viral infections.

In both clinical situations and the laboratory, researchers have been exploring ozone therapy as an effective procedure for treating cancer, and the findings on the positive effects of ozone at the cellular level are hope-ful. People with the disease have reported greater strength, less pain, and more appetite, and it seems to retard the rate of metastasis and tumor growth.

Ozone therapy in the management of HIV/AIDS is controversial, al-though small, promising studies in Canada and Cuba have shown that T-cell counts in patients with the disease have increased. Although most of the positive response has been anecdotal, in this sensitive area of test-ing new approaches to curing serious diseases, anecdotal research is often the beginning. Many with AIDS are more than willing to try controversial treatments because there is always the possibility of being able to extend their lives, or even be cured, and the anecdotal reports give them hope. Using ozone therapy, people with AIDS have increased their T-cell counts, seen their lymph nodes return to normal, and their diarrhea eliminated. Serious research still needs to be conducted, but as with all oxygen thera-pies, it is made difficult by strong opposition from the pharmaceutical industry. Their determination extends to holding off research on the devel-opment of potentially inexpensive, effective treatments because they know it could mean competition for their more expensive, often harsh, drugs.

Depending on the condition or illness being treated, ozone therapy, like the other oxygen therapies discussed here, is often used in combina-tion with other modalities. The physician's role as diagnostician is to use her or his expertise to determine how best to approach an illness or complaint. Having ozone therapy as one of the medical tools of the trade can only be beneficial to both patient and doctor.

There are three categories of conditions that could benefit from the use of ozone therapy, as follows:

1. Highly infected and badly healing wounds, as well as inflammatory conditions can benefit from ozone therapy. Abscesses and arthritis can be treated with minor autohemotherapy and, in certain situations, with major autohemotherapy. Orthopedic problems respond to ozone autohemotherapy, intramuscular injections, and intra-arterial injections. Anal fissures, molds and fungal infections, and skin conditions respond to treatment with external ozone and olive oil—ozonated oil therapy. Mouth inflammations, such as stomatitis or other dental problems, respond to treatment with ozonized water.

2. Circulatory disorders can benefit from treatment with various ozone therapies, particularly as they apply to problems of aging. Minor and major autohemotherapy can play an important role in treating allergies, arterial circulatory disorders, arteriosclerosis, asthma, gangrene, Parkinson's disease, Raynaud's disease, and even cancer.

3. Ozone therapy can be effective in viral diseases, particularly in the treatment of hepatitis with both major autohemotherapy and rectal insufflation. Herpes, too, all forms—genitalis, labialis, and zoster—respond to minor and major autohemotherapy.

I believe that ozone therapy, hyperbaric oxygen therapy, and hydrogen peroxide therapy, all designed to direct the flow of oxygen to the body to aid in healing, will find their public in the twenty-first century. There are indications of this in the public's interest and in the positive change within the medical community. The skepticism about the viability of less-known treatments is diminishing, and this could lead to a new era where ozone therapy would be as seriously respected a treatment option as drugs or surgery are now.

PART THREE

Photoluminescence—Ultraviolet Irradiation of Blood (UVIB)

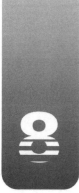

The Basics
of Ultraviolet
Irradiation
of Blood

*P*hotoluminescence, also known as ultraviolet irradiation of blood (UVIB), sounds like some mumbo-jumbo space-age or sci-fi treatment. It is, however, a remarkable therapeutic treatment that predates antibiotics. Not only is it effective in fighting infections, but it also produces few, if any, side effects in most people. And, like all the oxygen therapies discussed in this book, it is an approach to dealing with infections that is successfully used by thousands of people around the world. Unfortunately, it is virtually unknown by most Americans.

Discovered almost seventy years ago, UVIB was considered a preferred treatment for flu and allergies, significant for its ability to all but eliminate bacteria and viruses. However, its delivery process, as simple as it is, was still not as simple as taking a pill (and certainly not as commercially viable). This treatment consists of taking a small amount of blood— usually 60 cc to 120 cc—from the body, exposing it to ultraviolet light by passing it through a chamber, and then returning it to the body.

When antibiotics were developed in the 1940s, it didn't take long for entrepreneurs to build an industry on products that could be patented and marketed to physicians exclusively for them to dispense to patients on a prescription-only basis. Antibiotics were demonstrably effective treatments for infections, with so many seeming advantages that they pushed aside UVIB, despite its excellent track record in healing. Proponents touted antibiotics as the treatments that would wipe out infectious diseases forever. In the 1940s, the promotion and hype surrounding this new method made all other approaches seem old fashioned and, by implication, less effective. We now know, however, that many of the infectious organisms treated with these "wonder drugs" have developed deep resistances to them, and we continue to be plagued by both old and new strains that are more and more virulent—not to mention that antibiotics are useless against many toxins and all viruses.

UVIB was once called "the medicine of the future." It is my belief that the future for this form of treatment is now. Ultraviolet light was used early on to disinfect hospital rooms and surgical instruments, and to clean the air. It is still used for those purposes today. Currently, we are most familiar with its use to disinfect public toilet seats by exposing them to ultraviolet rays. Also, after the anthrax terrorist scares, Tom Ridge, Director of the Office of Homeland Security, and Postmaster General John Potter held a press briefing to discuss using ultraviolet light to sanitize the mail and protect the public against any trace amounts of anthrax that remained. When asked about installing sanitizing equipment, Potter said, referring to UV light, "It's a system that's safe. It's used on surgical equipment and medical supplies, so we're very comfortable that it's a safe technology." Perhaps, the terrorist attacks on September 11, 2001, and the threat of biological weapons will serve to revive interest in again using ultraviolet light as a treatment. I'm certain that publicizing UVIB's remarkable qualities will create a demand, if not for its immediate acceptance, then at least for further exploration. If a reexamination of ultraviolet light's healing potential stimulates interest in the process of irradiating blood, then physicians who are familiar with the process can make a safe, inexpensive treatment for people with bacterial and viral infections widely available. The use of biochemical weapons is a reality today; ways to counteract the plagues and the diseases they can cause are of paramount concern. I am not advocating that ultraviolet light therapy replace other methods of treatment, just that it should be offered as an option. Its capacity to destroy all surface viruses, bacteria, and fungi is impressive, but in my opinion, its most important contribution is what it can do within the body.

When ultraviolet light irradiates the blood, it empowers the immune system to kill invading organisms by stimulating that defense system, as well as the body's many enzyme systems, and thus returns the body to health very rapidly. The speed with which ultraviolet light therapies can kill biological agents is essential in a wartime environment. That speed can also be lifesaving in hospitals where viruses and bacteria thrive, and where patients with compromised immune systems can be infected on admission. Diseases like bacterial pneumonia demand immediate treatment. Moreover, with today's unique strains of bacteria and complicated new surgeries, the antibiotic needed to contain the microbe is often still in the laboratory. For me, it remains hard to believe that every hospital in this country is not equipped with the simple technology to deliver ultraviolet blood irradiation to patients—even if it is only on hand for use in emergencies.

HOW UVIB WORKS

How UVIB works has been one of the disadvantages of promoting this treatment for wider use, because although researchers have consistently observed remarkable changes in patients' health whenever the treatment was used, scientists have not been able to completely understand what happens to the blood reintroduced into the body after it has been exposed to ultraviolet light outside the body. In 1942, researcher Dr. Virgil Hancock found that toxins and viruses were rendered inactive, and bacteria growth was retarded; however, most interesting to Hancock was the noticeable increase in the blood's ability to carry more oxygen. Beyond that, other researchers observed UVIB's capacity to restore the chemical balance in the body, and its cumulative effect—each treatment enhances the results of the previous treatment, which is extremely important to the healing process. On the other hand, it has also been observed that too much ultraviolet radiation can produce depression and lessen resistance to bacterial infections, which points up the importance of educated medical monitoring of every treatment. This has been another problem. Because few physicians are familiar with ultraviolet irradiation of blood, few know how to use it to treat infections. Nor are they confident about its effectiveness or benefits, even though UVIB has consistently been shown to inactivate toxins in the body. Researchers also discovered that when viruses or infections received UVIB treatment early enough, 100 percent of the patients treated recovered completely.

Even in more recent times, I have found little written on how this therapy actually works. However, The Foundation for Light Therapy[1] has a plausible explanation. It states that photoluminescence "causes a chemical reaction in which the cell walls of the blood drawn from the body are pierced, killing the bacteria and virus, thereby . . . identifying them. The blood and the marked debris are then returned into the body . . . stimulating the immune system. The body's now excited, natural soldiers seek out and destroy the identified, diseased invaders. It is believed that, by destroying the bacteria in the treated sample of blood, an autogenous (self-generated) vaccine is produced. When this vaccine is coupled with the (light) energy previously absorbed by the treated blood, an induced secondary energy is released and the diseased cells in the patient's bloodstream are rapidly destroyed."

In his book, *Into the Light,* William Campbell Douglass said, "Fifty years have passed since George Miley and his colleagues attacked the foundations of modern medicine with photo-therapy. There is now a scientific explanation for the use of photo-irradiation in allergy. All toxic substances in the body have a fluorescence, including chemicals (tobacco), sick cells (cancer), and allergens (weeds, strawberries, or whatever you are allergic to). This fluorescence is, in effect, a marker which light energy targets for destruction. So when light energy (photons) is introduced directly into the blood, as in photo-oxidation, the recovery is often dramatic."

The October 2, 2000 issue of *US News & World Report* discussed the fact that "Scientists have now determined that the future for effective treatment with the least side effects is utilizing the body's own natural defenses." The interest in this approach to healing has caused researchers to explore the concept that light in various frequencies and intensities has the capacity to destroy bacteria, viruses, and fungi in blood by using the body's own natural ability not only to recognize, but also to kill, diseased cells. I believe that it is a very hopeful sign for those of us who have seen the results in patients treated with bio-oxidative therapies and UVIB.

UVIB—PAST TO PRESENT

Niels Ryberg Finsen began the work on ultraviolet radiation therapy in the late nineteenth century. His successful ultraviolet light treatments on 300 people with lupus brought him a Nobel Prize in 1903. In 1922, Kurt Naswitis, another pioneer, directly irradiated blood with UV light through a shunt. But it was not until 1928, when Emmett Knott irradiated the blood of a patient with a bloodstream infection after an abortion, that UVIB held out the promise of being a serious treatment for this common condition. The woman had not been expected to live, but UVIB returned her to complete health, and several years later, she was able to give birth to a healthy child. Emmett Knott and a fellow researcher, Virgil Hancock, presented breakthrough evidence of the effectiveness of photoluminescence in clinical use, and in 1928 Knott received a patent for a UV apparatus he built, subsequently receiving another patent in 1943 for changes to the equipment.[2]

During the 1940s, Dr. E. W. Rebbeck, Dr. George Miley, and Dr. Robert Olney all experimented with ultraviolet blood irradiation. "By June of 1942, 6,520 patients had been treated with ultraviolet therapy. Not only had the treatment worked nearly every time, it had done so in the complete absence of any harmful effects."[3]

Everyone working with UVIB became convinced that it was a remarkable treatment for infections. In the *American Journal of Bacteriology* (June 1943), Dr. George Miley reported that patients with viral pneumonia—to this day a serious problem to manage—who were treated with UVIB became symptom-free within twenty-four to seventy-six hours after only a single treatment. Coughs disappeared in less than a week, and chest x-rays revealed a complete clearing of the lungs, also within a week's time.

That such a successful treatment could be abandoned is a mystery to everyone, but in the 1950s, the introduction of new antibiotics pushed all oxygen and UVIB treatments into the background. In the 1970s, however, Russia began exploring UVIB again. About that same time, Dr. Richard L. Edelson at Yale University developed a new form of blood irradiation he called *photopheresis*—using UVIB to trigger chemotherapy. The method costs approximately $2,000 per treatment, but Yale University continues to treat about 900 patients per year using this therapy. According to The Foundation for Light Therapy, in the 1990s, Russian doctors used low-intensity lasers beamed directly into the blood for equivalent results.

In *Into the Light,* Dr. Douglass gives us a clue as to why, despite observable success, the treatment never achieved the visibility and use that it deserves. He says, "One of the most interesting things about the photoluminescent technique is that it does not kill bacteria directly. The fact is critical since only one twenty-fifth of the total blood volume is actually irradiated in the Knott technique. The procedure simply applies ultraviolet rays to the blood, utilizing a 'photon pump' (an ultraviolet light source) in an optimal dosage. Then, when reinjected, the irradiated blood somehow activates the rest of the body's defenses to attack the infection." He goes on to muse that, when the body metabolizes ultraviolet light, the healing effect is very subtle, and researchers could not confirm the results in laboratory settings outside the body—in petri dishes and test tubes—depriving them of any tangible evidence of success or failure. Moreover, the fact that such a small amount of irradiated blood visibly produced such dramatic results in the body did not make sense to researchers either. It seemed impossible, so rather than accept it as a possible treatment while studying it further, scientists rejected it, because, to them, understanding it was paramount to the scientific process. For them to apply it under those circumstances would be tantamount to admitting the limitations of medical science. Better to go with what you know, even if it has problems, they reasoned, than go with what you don't know, even though you risk nothing. So here we are again, some sixty years later, revisiting a treatment, reconsidering its potential to kill deadly infections better than the many establishment approaches that have been developed and used by conventional medicine in the intervening years.

Relative to this book, the fact that interests me most about UVIB is the increased oxygen in the veins. George Miley, a physician who used photoluminescence in his practice of medicine in the 1930s, observed a 58 percent increase in oxygen after ten minutes, followed by a 9 percent decrease within a half-hour, and then a 50 percent increase in venous oxygen anywhere from an hour to a month after a patient was injected. The additional oxygen was "in the plasma, the non-cellular portion of the blood." It was not due to "any increased oxygen-carrying capacity of the red blood cells because there was no rise in the red cell count to account for the oxygen increase."[4]

Dr. Miley also observed that when oxygen was present in the body, it neutralized bacterial toxins. He hypothesized that if UVIB was used in combination with intravenous hydrogen peroxide (see Chapter 6), which increases the amount of oxygen in the body, healing could happen even more quickly. Combining different oxygen treatments is now fundamental in my practice and in the practice of many complementary medical doctors. And even though we do not fully understand why higher oxygen levels outside the red blood cells help the healing process so immeasurably, the results are undeniable. Researchers other than Dr. Miley have noted that those treated with UVIB show a rise in the number of red blood cells, which, in fact, do also develop an increased capacity to carry oxygen. In my experience, the more oxygen I can get into patients, the faster their various symptoms are alleviated. So, faced with complicated physical conditions that have not responded to known drugs or surgical procedures, increasing the levels of oxygen in the body is a good place to start. Often, it is all that is needed to begin the upward climb back to health.

In the last forty years, serious research has been aimed at trying to understand why biological tissues irradiated with electromagnetic waves of different frequencies are affected. It has been a cross-disciplinary exploration, bringing together various sciences, including biology, electrical engineering, medicine, and physics. However, most of the existing controlled studies we cite to confirm the success of UVIB methodology date back to before 1950. Although this does not invalidate them, it does bring up questions about why research didn't continue and makes dismissal of the approach easy. The instant success of antibiotics doesn't appear to be enough of a reason for the cessation of testing, but still, all we have are old studies and anecdotal reports to make our case.

Having said this, it is important to note that the results of these old tests are very impressive. Mumps responded immediately after one treatment, with body temperatures back to normal in less than two days and swollen glands gone within five days. One hundred cases of skin infections caused by streptococcus—a deadly organism—were 100 percent cured with ultraviolet skin irradiation. Conditions like allergic asthma, botulism, bowel paralysis, diphtheria, tetanus, and many others respond rapidly to treatment. Even though there are other methods to treat such conditions, the speed with which ultraviolet irradiation of blood in the body and ultraviolet rays on the surface of the body work to affect improvement and cures needs to be examined.

The names of such doctors as Stephen B. Edelson, Virgil Hancock, Emmett Knott, and George Miley turn up time and again as innovators in this remarkable field. Dr. William Campbell Douglass's impressive case work in Uganda with AIDS patients, which will be discussed in Chapter 10, are among the most recent cases documented by a serious researcher.

UVIB IN THE UNITED STATES

In science, experiments that show such consistent results are generally given the benefit of a doubt and bring more funds to the research process, but it simply has not happened for UVIB in the United States. In places where medical treatment is less allied with politics (Russia, Eastern Europe, and Cuba, for example) and where money for healthcare is less available, there is a tendency to be pragmatic if the results are positive. So hyperbaric oxygen therapy, hydrogen peroxide therapy, and UVIB are not regarded as alternative therapies in these countries; they are considered practical medical treatments used by all physicians and recognized by the general public.

Our American culture, particularly in regard to medical treatment, has a technological perspective, and as consumers, we want instant cures, so our healthcare providers have spent decades promising us that new innovations in detection methods, pharmaceutical exploration, and surgical techniques will give us what we want. But I see patients every day who have tried everything conventional and are still sick. As practitioners of complementary medicine, we are in that unenviable position of practicing last-resort medicine. When nothing else works, people come to us. And more often than not, we can help. However, if we were a first-choice option, I believe help would come faster and the relative cost of treatment would be cheaper. Unfortunately, our treatments seem expensive because most insurance plans do not cover our approach to medicine, regardless of whether a patient is cured.

UVIB works quickly and the results are felt within a week or two, but there is no way around it; the treatment process requires time, and people are often inconvenienced because major medical centers do not offer the service. In the case of UVIB, the politics of medicine are a serious deterrent to wider exposure and use. From direct experience, I would say many people are unaware that treatments other than conventional ones even exist. If they were presented with explanations and a choice, they might very well ask for holistic care and even be willing to put up with a little inconvenience in order to feel better.

HOW I ADMINISTER ULTRAVIOLET IRRADIATION OF BLOOD

In treating colds or minor infections, pneumonia, or children's viral diseases, I generally use a pure quartz syringe in a continuous flow method to take out 1.5 milliliters of blood for every pound of body weight and expose it to ultraviolet light. I've found that a single treatment is often sufficient, and only occasionally does a condition require a second treatment.

The syringe is placed into a machine—Photolume II—designed to circulate ultraviolet light within. The syringe then rotates for three minutes of continuous exposure to ultraviolet light, as well as other wavelengths of the light spectrum. The syringe is now filled with irradiated blood, which I remove from the machine and reinject into the patient's arm. This method takes about thirty to forty-five minutes to complete.

Multiple Benefits of Ultraviolet Irradiation of Blood

*I*n all the literature on the oxygen therapies we deal with in this book, there is a frustration felt by those who have pioneered the treatments and carefully documented the case histories, the successful as well as unsuccessful outcomes. We realize that, as physicians practicing complementary medicine, we are regarded by mainstream medicine as unconventional at best. Some even uncharitably dismiss us as quacks. Such designations of our profession are unimportant, except for the fact that they make it more difficult for our approach to be seen by a greater population. My colleagues and I believe that the patient's welfare and return to health is the physician's responsibility, and that is what determines good medicine. And when a treatment doesn't work, the doctor must keep looking for other possible causes and pursuing other treatments for the illness or condition, which is why many of us place oxygen therapies among our most common treatments. They work more often than not for our patients, and they have fewer, if any, side effects more often than not. It is not an accident that our success rate for improvement and cure of many of the most troubling medical problems of our time is so high.

The medical profession has moved from whole-body concepts of healing to specialization, and several generations of physicians trained in this latter belief head departments and teach in medical schools. It's likely they suspect that oxygen therapies can't possibly be effective in treating such a wide range of conditions and diseases, because they probably feel that depth of experience and knowledge of a single illness or condition must *surely* have more validity. It is a difficult mindset for both patients and doctors to overcome. How is it possible that a treatment that can cure shingles—something conventional doctors regard as chronic—can also be used to dramatically improve the symptoms of AIDS. It is not only possible, it happens every day someplace in the world. And the number of different chronic and disease states that respond to this particular medical approach is astonishing, even to me who understands the principles and has seen patients' health improve dramatically. Unfortunately, instead of such successes stimulating interest and curiosity, I think they tend to make many people skeptical. It is illogical, but many people today feel protected and comfortable when a specialized drug or procedure exists for their condition or disease alone. Treatments with more general application are often suspect.

It is frustrating to try and explain to a skeptical patient that, if all the specialized procedures, drugs, and treatments they have tried for their condition have not worked, one more try—with evidence to back up its effectiveness, and with no side effects—should be risked. It is only an emotional risk, moreover, because no physical harm will occur. And more important, there is the great possibility of feeling better. I want to say, risk getting well, but I believe the patient is responsible for making his or her own healthcare decisions, and I refrain from promoting one treatment over another. My philosophy is to offer all the options for consideration, make a recommendation, and leave open the possibility that if we don't agree, the patient might reconsider at a different time. The impetus for a change of mind is different in everyone, and a doctor knows more clearly than anyone that a patient must be fully ready for a treatment or procedure. Healing is a very individual process.

Jim Henson, the creator of the Muppets, was taken ill with streptococcus A and died very quickly from the virulent toxin it produced. It would not respond to any known antibiotic. If the hospital had been equipped to treat Henson with photoluminescence, proven to kill the toxin within hours, he might have lived.[1] And there was medical precedent for this treatment. A landmark case, reported by Dr. George Miley in the June 1944 issue of the *American Journal of Surgery*, dealt with the complete recovery of nine consecutive patients from *Staphylococcus a. septicemia*. What happened in the intervening years to allow such an effective treatment to be withheld by, or unknown to, Henson's doctors who must have known how seriously ill he was? If they had known about photoluminescence, wouldn't it have been worth trying it in order to save his life?

Bronchial asthma, a chronic allergic condition, threatens the well-being of thousands of people commonly treated with inhalers—injections of epinephrine and other medications—and sometimes even with surgery. In the late 1930s and the 1940s, George Miley studied eighty patients with the illness who were not responding to any treatment. Ultraviolet irradiation of blood treatments were administered every four to six weeks, and the symptoms improved in all but eleven people. Eventually, those in the study needed only a single treatment every eight to ten weeks. Regarding the outcome of the eleven patients who did not improve, it is noted that, unlike today, intravenous hydrogen peroxide was not regularly used as a support treatment to increase the oxygen level.

Louise's Many Health Problems

When Louise came to my office after listening to my radio program, she said, "I just don't feel well. I never feel well." It's the most common complaint I hear, and when I hear it, I know it's the beginning of solving another mystery. She'd had medical consultations before, she said, but nothing had changed. After some diagnostic testing—a six-hour urine test for heavy metal toxicity, blood tests, and stool analysis—we discovered that she had mercury toxicity, a mycoplasma infection, and arthritis. She was having some dental work done when she consulted with us and silver amalgam showed in the tests, so we suggested a follow-up with a biological dentist.

I prescribed medications, supplements, and vitamins, and 250 grams of DMSA (dimercapto-succinic acid) chelation every other day. Chelation aids in the cellular detoxification of heavy metals. But I knew from the test results that the core treatment for her various problems should be ultraviolet irradiation of blood (UVIB). And I was right. After ten UVIB treatments, Louise could say, "I feel better." And after ten more sessions, a total of twenty, her blood tests for mercury toxicity and the mycoplasma infection were negative and her general health was completely improved. She now receives UVIB treatments on a maintenance basis.

The generalized sense of not feeling well that doesn't go away is what prompts most patients to seek out complementary physicians. Sometimes, as with Louise, it is a combination of chronic health problems and potential disease states that add up to not being able to live life fully and often precede the onset of serious illness.

Dr. Robert Olney, one of the pioneers of photoluminescence, believed strongly that it could wipe out cancer and serious infectious diseases. In the 1960s, the results of his studies using ultraviolet irradiation of blood for five people with cancer were published. The conditions treated included malignant melanoma, metastatic colon cancer, two cases of thyroid cancer, and uterine cancer, and all five people recovered with ultraviolet irradiation of blood.

Dr. William Douglass has also successfully treated bone and brain cancers, secondary to breast and stomach cancers, with ultraviolet irradiation of blood. The symptoms of the woman with brain cancer included severe headaches, weight loss, hair loss, and nausea, which were all eliminated. A brain scan showed there was no further growth, demonstrating that the treatment stopped the advance of the cancer. Once she stopped the therapy, however, her condition deteriorated, and Dr. Douglass notes that he was never able to "regain the lost ground . . . and she died from respiratory arrest." Dr. Douglass notes that nobody has ever cured metastatic brain cancer, and although he does not claim a successful cure, his methods extended the woman's life and vastly improved the quality of it.

Blood poisoning—septicemia—responds dramatically to treatment with photoluminescence. Sometimes the headaches, muscle aches, and

Finding the Right Complementary Care

Jose, a sixty-two-year-old Hispanic man who had little success with conventional medicine, had been researching complementary and alternative approaches to his illness, chronic hepatitis C. He learned about the range of services at The CAM Institute for Integrative Therapies, and that is what convinced him to become a patient. Among the services, the institute offers UVIB. He had a history of this persistent illness and had previously taken interferon and even participated in an experimental study for hepatitis C before coming to see me. I recommended UVIB, and after several treatments, his liver function tests showed improvement, encouraging us to continue in this direction. After four months and fourteen UVIB treatments, Jose's liver functioning improved by almost 50 percent. Although his chronic condition has not been eliminated, the functioning of his liver has greatly improved.

other pains disappear in as short a time as ten minutes. A serious cases of peritonitis was once cured in twenty-eight hours.[2]

Dr. Douglass's book *Into the Light*—one of the very few dealing with photoluminescence—outlines the details of various cases, and I have relied on his research to back up my own observations of results while treating patients with UVIB.

I firmly believe there is a future for photoluminescence in helping to end the serious diseases, such as cancer and HIV/AIDS, that have plagued us during the latter half of the twentieth century and on into this one. As a working physician, I am grateful to be able to use this treatment, knowing it gives me the means to help improve the ordinary lives of people whose day-to-day illnesses, conditions, and health problems are so debilitating, sap our energy, keep us from our jobs, and prevent us from enjoying life. Most of the people I see come to my office with common ailments, such as allergies, bronchitis, candidiasis, depressed immune system, flu, herpes, Lyme disease, or yeast infections. And these are all conditions I can manage with photoluminescence, as well as with the other oxygen therapies discussed in this book. To achieve total health, I may additionally recommend changes in diet, chelation therapy, or vitamin therapy. Acupuncture, too, is a useful and effective treatment. Again, I emphasize that an individual treatment program is often a combination of several modalities working together to return a person to health.

Saving Lives with Ultraviolet Irradiation of Blood

I want to be careful not to overstate the case for oxygen therapies and, in particular, ultraviolet irradiation of blood because I believe so strongly in its value. Frankly, many of us who practice these complementary methods have such remarkable success in treating our patients and improving their health that we cannot believe we are so disregarded by mainstream medicine, and, to compensate, we are sometimes guilty of selling the truth when we know that simply telling it should suffice. UVIB, or photoluminescence, is all I have been telling you it is, but it is currently difficult for most people to find access to the treatment. It is also not as easy as taking a pill, though, on the other hand, a pill cannot accomplish what UVIB can. It demands time to undergo the procedure, requires taking blood, and is not inexpensive (each treatment at my center ranges from $175–$200). And, as I stated in the beginning of this part, although this therapy sounds like some space-age futuristic medicine, the delivery method is not very sexy, nor very technological. It has remained pretty much the same since its development. The machinery does not look like shiny CAT scan equipment, nor is it necessary to perform the procedure in a sterile operating room. The process is, in fact, unprepossessing. But it is able to do something right now that other existing approaches to treating infectious diseases have yet to do as successfully, and that is to destroy all those disease-causing viruses and bacteria in the body—including the new ones surfacing every day—with no side effects.

In the last chapter, we discussed the multiple benefits of ultraviolet irradiation of blood for many chronic conditions and diseases. These conditions and ailments—allergies, asthma, cancer, gingivitis, hepatitis, herpes,

111

pneumonia, and so on—affect us, members of our families, our friends, and our colleagues. However, the story of Dr. William Douglass's eight-week experience in Uganda treating patients who had contracted AIDS caused by HIV with photoluminescence underlines the importance of this treatment and the urgent need to make it available to the world as soon as possible. The problem with HIV/AIDS is that "the lymphatic system serves as the primary reservoir for the virus, which can destroy the immune system within two to ten or more years. Individuals infected with HIV may not be symptomatic for years, while others progress rapidly."[1] An epidemic may be in the making before people are even aware that it is happening.

HIV/AIDS is spreading around the world at an epidemic rate. Most current drug regimens cannot work quickly enough, if at all, to stem the tide. If the drugs are available, those receiving them must be able to follow through on taking accurate doses of them, according to a time schedule that is often inconvenient. It is overwhelming, even to people who are used to a Western medical approach, but in less developed countries, people are simply confused by what is required of them and are often unable to continue the program. Even if they can manage to sort out the treatment routine, the side effects of these HIV/AIDS drugs are serious. Added to all this is the high cost. Even when the Western pharmaceutical companies cut the price, drastically by their standards, it remains very high for most of the world's populations.

HIV/AIDS AND UVIB CASE STUDIES

In 1989, Dr. Douglass was permitted by the Ugandan government to set up a clinic primarily to treat HIV/AIDS with hydrogen peroxide therapy and photoluminescence. Dr. Douglass believed Uganda was a good place to begin this work because the leadership of the country put politics aside and openly revealed that it was facing a monumental health problem that could bring a halt to its functioning as a society if something was not done. In Dr. Douglass's 1993 book, *Into the Light,* he quoted statistics that were frightening even then. "In 1983, seventeen cases were reported, in 1984, twenty-nine cases, in 1987, there were 1,138 cases, and the case load is rapidly increasing." He said that if the numbers continued to increase at that pace, they could expect that, by the millennium, half of all Uganda's citizens could be affected by the virus—a statistic that has, unfortunately, become true.

In Dr. Douglass's case histories, he reported that the most common symptoms were alleviated within weeks—fevers disappeared, diarrhea ended, rashes cleared up, appetites returned, weight gain occurred, and the people returned to work. In some cases, however, the patients got better in the short run but then went downhill. The health of some patients with other diseases and conditions in addition to HIV/AIDS, or those who do not continue treatments, failed.

The case studies of the small sample of patients Dr. Douglass treated were very hopeful. The fact is, however, that these cases continue to be regarded as anecdotal and cannot represent enough of a sample to bring the kind of serious attention to the treatment that could spur the scientific community to encourage its use on a mass scale. In the chapter of his book that discusses his case studies from Africa, Dr. Douglass says something that clearly expresses the reason for our frustration as complementary physicians, namely that, even with experience and personal case histories to prove the value of a treatment, we simply cannot find a way to make it available to everyone who needs it.

"Today, (1994) three years after (these) cases were treated, dramatic changes have occurred in the African clinic," says Dr. Douglass. "Word of the remarkable improvements seen in terminally ill patients with 'slim' (another name for AIDS, which causes serious weight loss) has traveled across the country and the clinic is inundated with patients. Record-keeping and laboratory monitoring is practically non-existent but patients look only for results and don't care a banana about T cells and P-24 counts. You don't have to be a microbiologist to see that the treatment is working. When Jobwa comes home with a thirty-pound weight gain and his skin rot is gone, the family has seen enough. The brothers, sisters, aunts, and uncles lined up at the clinic. A twenty-four-hour wait doesn't matter; they'll pitch a tent in the front yard."

And, as is true for all those affected, talk of T cells and schedules and side effects are just too many words. They only want to feel better and not be sick, even for a little while, and we as doctors want the same thing for them. But the reality is that we have to curb our impatience and get the documentation in whatever way we can. We believe that the more information we can deliver to the public about these treatments, the more convincing we can be about their value, then more doctors may come around to considering their effectiveness and ask for more studies confirming our experience with the treatments. It is difficult for laypeople to comprehend the expense involved in documenting the vast numbers of case histories needed to validate a treatment. Meanwhile, we can only treat patients who know of the treatment or are referred to us by physicians who are enlightened or have run out of conventional procedures. This frustrates us because we know that we can save countless numbers of lives and improve the health of millions of people with UVIB.

UVIB IN RUSSIA

My Russian medical training has given me confidence in UVIB that would have been difficult for doctors in the United States to achieve. The work of Emmett Knott and the other innovators in the early twentieth century was well known to us in Russia as a safe, effective treatment, and it has been in use for more than thirty years now. Even conservative Russian physicians have accepted it, perhaps because the financial underpinnings of Russian medicine were weak, and UVIB was inexpensive and effective. Under those circumstances, the fact that it was unconventional could be overlooked. In the early years, UVIB was used mostly as an antimicrobial agent, but we realized very quickly that it could be used to treat a variety of pathological conditions.

In his 1991 visit to Russia, Dr. Douglass spoke admiringly about surgeons Kutushev and Chalenko of the City Center for the Fotomodification of Blood in St. Petersburg. Here, the use of UVIB was said to have cut in half the "number of complications, and the necessity to use antibiotics in severe trauma cases." Beyond that, Douglass noted that they had treated

The Foundation for Light Therapy

The Foundation for Light Therapy is providing photoluminescence and other oxidative medical therapies in certain African countries. They reported that their first mission to Africa was considered "miraculous" by those who witnessed their successes. "The Foundation has compiled extensive evidence that further development and experimentation with these technologies will save millions of lives. The Foundation intends to enlist the expertise of medical professionals, institutions, organizations, and specialists to help further the development of these promising treatments." (Mission of the Foundation) more than 3,000 patients using UVIB. If such success had been achieved in the United States, some savvy medical reporter would have done a story on it for the television networks and a flurry of interest would have followed. But despite Dr. Douglass's enthusiasm and his urgent demands for consideration of the treatment, UVIB has passed into the twenty-first century virtually unnoticed. What is hopeful to me, however, is that UVIB continues to be practiced. Those who have been successfully treated develop an underground support system, a word-of-mouth advertising campaign that becomes more effective as UVIB continues to cure what ails them and makes them feel better. If conventional treatments had succeeded, there would have been no need to seek further. To date, our timing may have been off, but I am certain that when UVIB is effectively used in a high-profile situation, the media will take notice and, before we know it, the African and Russian successes will be "discovered" and the U.S. demand for research will begin.

In Russia, UVIB treatment for burns is worth noting. The work of Dr. V. M. Novopolzev's team from Mordovsky University in Saransk has been particularly successful, according to Douglass. In 1992, they reported "sixteen cases of severe third-degree burns, some of them covering as much as 69 percent of the body surface." The following are the surgeons' observations from the Saransk medical conference, held in 1992 in Russia, as reported by Dr. Douglass in *Into the Light.*

1. The patients' "common state" improved almost immediately after re-infusion of the UV-irradiated blood. Their appetites also improved markedly.

2. The severe pain subsided and they were able to stop injections of narcotics in many of the patients.

3. Because of these favorable clinical changes, the patients would often fall into a deep sleep for the first time since their burn accidents.

4. The protein content of the blood plasma usually increased after the first infusion of irradiated blood—a very good sign in burn patients, as protein loss is one of the major problems in these cases.

The Russian doctors and researchers are continuing their clinical studies involving the use of UVIB in an entire range of medical disciplines, including all the infectious diseases, cardiovascular illnesses, dermatology, gynecology, immunology, and neurology. It is difficult for Americans to understand that these "medical successes" in Russia are often achieved in environments that are primitive by Western medical standards. Even facing a hopeless diagnosis from their own physicians, most people in the United States would be reluctant to seek help in such circumstances. I am not suggesting that they do, either, because it is not necessary. In the relatively few places where UVIB treatment is available here, the treatments are executed in clean, safe, clinical surroundings, yet the unfamiliar nature of UVIB still keeps patients and their physicians wary about exploring this effective approach to better health.

PART FOUR

The Oxygen Therapies and How They Work Together

The Remarkable
Oxygen Therapies

*O*nly in an environmentally balanced Garden of Eden would human beings be able to take in the exact amount of oxygen, fruits, vegetables, and pure water to ideally supplement our daily oxygen needs in order to keep our bodies healthy. In such a world, energy would always be high and the ability to ward off illness would be like second nature. But this is the twenty-first century. The fact is, our air and water are compromised and our food supply lacks nutrients.

Furthermore, we have sacrificed much of what is natural in our environment in order to advance our society and achieve technological superiority. Without our health, these advancements and achievements pale in importance, and it becomes difficult to maintain our dreams or to realize the future, so the pursuit of health is fundamental to our personal happiness and societal success. Chronic conditions and lifestyle illnesses— those aggravated by inadequate diets and lack of exercise, smoking, drinking, and stress, as well as those from circumstances we do not control—can be alleviated, improved, and even cured by getting enough oxygen into our bodies and revitalizing our cells. When we combine this effort to get the oxygen we need with a proper diet, appropriate physical exercise, vitamins and herbs to build our bodies, and hands-on therapies, such as massage or acupuncture when necessary, we have a program that maximizes our health.

But first, we need to focus on our bodies and understand that staying healthy demands as much of us as any other goal we have for ourselves. This accomplishment makes all others possible. It has been my experience, however, that most people today live in their heads and simply allow their bodies to trail along, driven by that super-energized, ever-active brain. But the head has a body, and ideally it should all work together.

Holistic medicine is focused on the whole body. It is the only medicine that begins by using natural sources as medicine—the basics of what human beings need to survive on this earth in the best possible way: pure oxygen, pure water, nutritious organic food, natural herbs and vitamins from natural sources, and appropriate physical exercise. We begin by treating the patient with the basics, and then we add treatments that use the body's own resources, such as acupuncture, chelation, chiropractic, or massage, to heal itself. As our natural resources become degraded, illnesses result, and our job as complementary physicians becomes more difficult. We have to teach our patients how to upgrade their bodies by supplementing what today's life does not easily provide. Natural treatments and natural medicine bypass chemicals, and when possible, we believe patients should avoid surgery. However, as complementary physicians we are fortunate. When stronger means are needed to improve a condition, we can prescribe pharmaceuticals and suggest other medical intervention because, by that time, we know our patient and what is needed for her or his optimum health.

Food with its nutrients intact is healing. I design diets to alleviate the allergies and chronic illnesses that conventional physicians try to treat with drugs. Pure water is healing, and I tell every single patient I see that it is an essential basic in their health routine. Physical movement is healing, and every patient of mine is aware that regular exercise is basic to health.

Of all the basic needs, however, oxygen is by far the most crucial for human beings. The purer the air we breathe, the healthier our bodies remain. But when used appropriately, oxygen's most underrated quality is its power to heal human bodies. Like food and water, the healing qualities work continually in our bodies, but when our bodies become unbalanced and our physical function gets distorted, additional oxygen can be used to restore health. Throughout this book, I have tried to show that the therapeutic infusion of oxygen into the body often results in miraculous disappearance of symptoms. But today's tenacious diseases, many simply the result of our contemporary life, are not about to disappear.

In my many years of medical practice, I have discovered that, as significant as a single oxygen therapy can be in improving a condition, when you combine it with one, or even two, other oxygen therapies, you multiply the benefits and bring about quicker improvements and cures.

Hyperbaric oxygen therapy alone is very effective. However, even though hyperbaric chambers are available in most hospitals, only a few conditions will be paid for by insurance, and most hospitals will not make the chambers available for the many diseases and conditions I know can be improved with this therapy. (See Appendix A for a listing of hyperbaric oxygen therapy centers by state.) Hyperbaric oxygen therapy also complements other bio-oxidative therapies—hydrogen peroxide therapy, ozone therapy, ultraviolet irradiation of blood—and if you can find a facility that is equipped to use all of these therapies, your choices for staying healthy are maximized.

As discussed, hydrogen peroxide therapy alone is also very effective in treating a myriad of conditions, and in many instances, it is all that is needed to rebalance the body. But in combination with hyperbaric oxygen therapy, ozone therapy, or ultraviolet irradiation of blood, long-term remission can become an easy reality in serious illnesses such as HIV/ AIDS. In his book *Oxygen Healing Therapies,* Nathaniel Altman says that investigations are taking place to determine the most effective combinations for treating HIV/AIDS. In addition to the bio-oxidative therapies, other approaches, such as Chinese herbs, or oral alpha interferon may be part of the mix. He lists an organization called Keep Hope Alive as a source to contact for the most recent information on useful combinations of approaches.

In my own practice, I have found that hyperbaric oxygen therapy, in combination with hydrogen peroxide therapy, is a highly effective treatment approach for cerebral palsy, chronic fatigue syndrome, immune deficiency syndrome, improving or stabilizing multiple sclerosis, memory loss due to mini-strokes (vascular dementia), and peripheral vascular disease (PVD), just to name a few. I have even found that Down syndrome, for which conventional medicine has few treatments to improve the symptoms, responds to oxygen treatment. As with all the oxygen therapies, we do not talk about cure (although, in fact, many cures are achieved), but in almost all the cases where I have prescribed oxygen therapies, singly or in combination, they have significantly improved my patients' conditions, sometimes slowly, sometimes dramatically. Is it any wonder that I prescribe them so often?

In 1997, at the Eighth International Conference on Bio-Oxidative Medicine in Anchorage, Alaska, Dr. Kenneth Bock presented a paper on his successful treatment of more than 1,000 patients with Lyme disease by combining complementary approaches. Hydrogen peroxide, hyperbaric oxygen, herbs, and nutritional supplements all worked together to eliminate the serious effects of the disease.

In my book *Why Can't I Remember?*, I deal with the whole question of memory loss, something most healthy people assume is a natural part of the aging process. Not so. Through oxidation therapies, such as hydrogen peroxide therapy, hyperbaric oxygen therapy, and ozone therapy—alone or in some combination—oxygen supplies are increased in the blood and tissues. As stated in *Why Can't I Remember?*, "They strengthen the red blood cells that feed memory and they help keep the membranes surrounding memory cells flexible for nutrient absorption. In addition, oxygen therapies help improve the body's own enzyme processes that fight brain aging. They also speed up energy production from sugar in the blood and neurons. Finally, these therapies increase oxygen levels in memory tissue." The more oxygen we can get to the brain, the clearer we think, and the more functional our memory. Combining oxygen therapies maximizes the amount of oxygen our bodies receive, and this is a good thing. Who among us approaching middle age has not wondered if there was anything we could do to improve our memories. Even ginkgo biloba, despite its claims, has little muscle up against any of the oxygen therapies.

The African studies I discussed in Chapter 10 underline the value of combining hydrogen peroxide therapy with ultraviolet irradiation of blood in an effort to stem the tide of HIV/AIDS. Many of the case histories cited by Dr. William Douglass involved a combination of oxygen treatments— again, getting as much oxygen to the affected cells as quickly as possible.

This book has focused primarily on using oxygen therapies to treat illness, disease, or abnormal body functioning. But I believe that the role of the complementary physician has two facets. The first is that of the conventional doctor to whom you go as a patient because you are ill, or fear something is going wrong in your body. The reason for this is simple. It's how mainstream medicine is set up. And today it is even more complicated. If you can determine what part of your body is involved, you go to a specialist, so it is only natural to assume that complementary medicine operates on that same model. But it doesn't. When you come to see us, you have to disabuse yourself of the specialist concept because we believe the body must be seen as a whole entity first. So when you come to us for medical consultation, you can use us as conventional doctors, but know, also, that we will explore the status of the whole body as it connects to the specific, rather than the other way around.

The second role of the complementary physician is health maintenance, which is a prime motive in complementary medicine. I think of using oxygen therapies to maintain *maximum* functioning in healthy people. Helping healthy people remain healthy, in much the same way a chiropractor, a dentist, a massage therapist, or a psychiatrist does, is what I see as an ideal role for complementary physicians. If we are a regular part of your health maintenance, we can help enhance your well-being. The human body is a changing, evolving entity. Health fluctuates as outside conditions change, as stresses mount and recede, as colds and viral symptoms develop from normal exposure to other people. Our sensitivity to the energies of our specific environments, the people we work and live with, combined with our physical response to these factors, determines the state of our health. And so it makes total sense to have a continuing relationship with a professional who monitors your health, recommends changes to your normal routine, and also cares for you when you are ill.

Just as you exercise daily on your own, or at the gym with your trainer, in order to maintain your strength—just as you get periodic adjustments from your chiropractor, or relieve muscle tension by getting a massage—seeing your complementary physician three or four times a year for various oxygen therapies, nutritional updates, and chelation therapy to clear out the sludge in your blood vessels is health maintenance. These are all alternative ways to strengthen your immune system so your body can fight minor illnesses quickly and prevent the development of serious disease. And how about scheduling a monthly HBOT treatment to prevent burn-outs? Or how about getting a hydrogen peroxide treatment at the height of the flu season? We call this preventive medicine, but complementary medicine has moved into the twenty-first century, and now we actively work to sustain health rather than simply prevent disease. It is not a small distinction.

The cost of complementary medicine over a year's time is minor. The visits are covered by most insurance companies, or Medicare, even though oxygen therapies and other alternative treatments may not be. Ask your complementary physician for his or her recommendation on using oxygen as a health maintenance treatment, in combination with a high-quality diet and regular exercise.

To repeat, the more oxygen that reaches your body's cellular structure, the more vital your body will be. Be aware that our food, our water, and our air are the natural sources of oxygen. That awareness will help us get the most from them by choosing wisely and by being conscious of how important these choices are. Beyond that, we need to know it may not be enough to sustain our health. Oxygen therapies, alone and working together, can supplement the oxygen we get naturally; they have the capacity to maintain our bodies and, more important, to strengthen the weaknesses, heal the illnesses, and repair the body. Oxygen is the master healer. We must not take it for granted.

Conclusion

WIDENING THE HORIZONS FOR MEDICINE IN THE TWENTY-FIRST CENTURY

*A*n overview of American medicine during the last twenty years would surely point to exceptional progress in the areas of technologically advanced diagnostic equipment, followed by groundbreaking pharmaceutical research, and, finally, by the development of microsurgical techniques aided by computer. There is no denying their combined importance in treating disease by conventional means or as support to any complementary medical practice. Magnetic resonance imaging (MRI), CT scans, and improvements in mammography have been able to help doctors diagnose illnesses much earlier than was possible in years past. Advanced drug treatments, particularly in the area of chemotherapy for the treatment of cancer, have improved the chances for increased survival but, of course, not without side effects. And the possibility of performing intricate surgery inside the body accurately, subjecting the patient to far less pain and anger, and less recovery time, is changing the nature of surgery.

But what has changed medicine most, in my opinion, has happened in the past quarter century And that is the attitudinal change, by ordinary women and men, toward health and medical care, a shift that I believe has opened the door to the health direction of the future—complementary medicine. Not since the early 1920s have so many people shown an interest in a medical philosophy that emphasizes the body's ability to heal itself in combination with current medical knowledge and technology.

In March 2002, the Department of Continuing Education at Harvard Medical School offered a seminar on "Complementary and Integrative Medicine, State of the Science and Clinical Applications." When one of the premier medical schools in the United States develops a course in my specialization, I know we are no longer on the far fringe of medicine. This course was developed, in part, with grants from some partners unusual for Harvard, which include The Cambridge Muscular Therapy Institute, The New England School of Acupuncture, The New York Chiropractic College, and The National Center for Complementary and Alternative Medicine, National Institutes of Health, among others. The program presented is still middle-of-the-road complementary medicine, dealing with known quantities, such as acupuncture, chiropractic, dietary supplements, herbs, and therapeutic massage, as well as workshops dealing with integrative/ complementary medical approaches to disease areas such as cancer, cardiology, and low back pain. There were also presentations and workshops devoted to the business of medicine, discussing liability and malpractice, as well as advising patients. Although there is still a very long way to go before complementary goes mainstream, seminars such as this make me hopeful.

The growing interest in complementary and integrative medicine began as a deep discontentment and frustration with the existing system, and very slowly escalated into anger. Technological advancements were primarily available to private patients and seemed to discriminate against people unable to pay for them. Managed care further alienated people. The impersonal, financially driven bureaucracy seemed patently unfair to most. And many experienced physicians, tired of the paperwork and the expense of running an office to meet corporate needs, threw up their hands, closed their offices, and left the profession, creating a void in the number of doctors needed to meet patient demand. Fewer students applied to nursing schools, and understaffed hospitals turned to inexperienced aides and orderlies to try and bridge the gap. We all know what happened as a result—a decline in care, a lack of personal attention from physicians, and numerous mistakes that threaten patient health.

It is no wonder that many people simply reached their levels of tolerance and began looking around for something else. And so the natural health movement, with its emphasis on prevention, natural medicine, and self-empowerment found itself rediscovered in the 1980s and 1990s. Although more visible earlier in the twentieth century, as previously mentioned, the movement never completely disappeared, but had been very slowly gaining advocates as technological medicine was discovered to be both fallible and expensive. The traditional concepts of organic food, pure air and water, herbs, vitamins, and hands-on bodywork, were embraced by health writers and journalists as if they were brand new. Health and healthcare became fashionable, particularly because the natural health movement was about far more than treating illness. It was about body consciousness, preventing illness and disease, feeling better, looking better, and basically taking responsibility for your own body and its health, instead of just passively having your medical decisions made for you. Immigrants arriving from the Far East—Japan, China, and India—brought with them concepts that connected body and mind. This struck a chord in the national consciousness and opened our minds to the possibility of viable alternatives to drugs and surgery. We had a choice. People fed up with the impersonal, often rude, behavior of healthcare workers and the long waits in doctors' offices began to consider such seemingly esoteric treatments as Chinese herbal medicine, Japanese shiatsu massage therapy, Ayurvedic medicine from India, and American Indian herbs. And many of them became converts to the whole idea of body/mind medicine, combining disciplines from many cultures. But, more important, they felt comfortable structuring a natural health program for themselves.

Feeling free to make their own decisions, Americans actively sought information in books and magazines, and from the Internet when it came along, to learn about their specific concerns. The cult of rigid medical authority was beginning to break down. If they felt better, it made them feel more confident about continuing to pursue approaches to health that were frowned on by conventional doctors. They were equally confident about choosing or refusing a surgical procedure or a drug. The vitamin, herb, and health-products industries grew dramatically. People were learning to treat themselves when they had colds, the flu, or minor illnesses, using supplements and herbs such as vitamin C, echinacea, goldenseal, and CoQ_{10}, and only going to a doctor when self-medication was not working. Threatened, the medical bureaucracy responded, using their powerful resources to restrict the effectiveness of herbs and supplements, but the public fought back because it had grown used to getting results from self-treatment. It is a continuing battle, however, and until the medical community stops insisting on putting their financial priorities over their patients' priorities, we will need to be watchful of any interest groups that want to deny ordinary people access to natural health aids.

Naturally, any approach to healthcare that is so loosely structured is bound to attract a few charlatans, though even traditional medicine has also seen its share of charlatans in the form of unlicensed doctors practicing openly, and badly, in America's communities. But I want to assure you that the vast majority of complementary physicians are professionals, educated not only in medicine, with degrees from established universities, but also schooled, formally and informally (sometimes in apprenticeships), in herbal medicine and folk traditions, as well as in alternative treatments not embraced by mainstream medicine—the oxygen therapies, for example. We look like your own physicians, and we work in clinical surroundings. But there the similarity ends.

Most important for the evolution of complementary medicine, the people discovered that they liked the philosophical basis of natural medicine: That human beings are individuals with different biochemical, emotional, physiological, and psychological components that together can determine their state of health. Natural medicine respected their intuitive belief that making a diagnosis demanded time from the doctor to get to know a patient. And when enough people wanted the same things, a movement was in the making.

Some statistics drawn from the course catalog to the Harvard University seminar on Complementary and Integrative Medicine[1] prove there is a deep reservoir of interest on the part of the general public for the services of complementary physicians and practitioners and also a willingness to buy products that are advertised to them directly or prescribed by their physicians. These studies are as follows:

"Between 1990 and 1997:

1. The prevalence of CAM (complementary/alternative medicine) use increased by 25 percent, from 33.8 percent in 1990 to 42.1 percent in 1997.

2. The prevalence of herbal remedy use increased by 380 percent.

3. The prevalence of high-dose vitamin use increased by 130 percent.

4. The total number of visits to CAM providers increased by 47 percent, from 427 million in 1990 to 629 million in 1997.

5. The total visits to CAM providers (629 million) exceeded total visits to all primary care physicians (386 million) in 1997.

6. In 1997, adults made an estimated 33 million office visits to professionals for advice regarding the use of herbs and high-dose vitamins.

7. Estimated expenditures for CAM professional services increased by 45 percent, exclusive of inflation, and were estimated at $21.2 billion dollars in 1997.

8. In 1997, an estimated 15 million adults took prescription medications concurrently with herbal remedies and/or high-dose vitamins. These individuals are therefore at risk for adverse drug-herb or drug-supplement interactions.

9. Current use of CAM services is likely to under-represent utilization patterns if insurance coverage for CAM therapies increases in the future."

Most people—regardless of whether they seek conventional or alternative healthcare—now believe that what you eat and how you cook is important to a healthy body. They know that stress is a factor in illness and disease and that family medical history is important. They want what they have always wanted in a doctor, but had given up hope of finding—a caring woman or man who is challenged by the desire to make people feel better and get well, a doctor who knows and accepts that patients also bear some of the responsibility for healing. A change in attitudes and expectations for medicine has arrived, and there will be even more change in the twenty-first century.

The challenge for us as complementary physicians is to find more young physicians to join our ranks. Although there is a rapidly growing demand for our kind of medicine, there are too few of us at the present time. We are left just as shorthanded as our more conventional colleagues. We need more doctors who are open-minded in their approach to medicine, who use common sense, intuition, and practical experience in their treatment of patients. Physicians are not gods; they are partners in their patient's journey in healthcare. They share equal responsibility for physical improvements and enjoy equal success at their achievements.

I am optimistic about the possibility of complementary and establishment medicine joining ranks. Medical schools will have to change curriculums. Elective courses in alternative medicine are already offered in many colleges, but as the demand for *unconventional* treatment (so termed

by today's biases) grows more insistent, I know that once-elective courses will have to become required courses, and that will make alternative
medicine, as it exists today, more professional. The medical degree of the
future will ensure that most doctors know the entire range of therapies,
treatments, and possibilities—conventional and complementary. Ideally,
a world medical curriculum will be taught in schools, one encompassing
the ancient alternative practices of Ayurvedic medicine, Chinese medicine, and Tibetan medicine, and the more recent alternative therapies
(oxygen or chelation, for example), along with technologically driven
Western diagnostic techniques, pharmaceuticals, and advanced surgical
techniques. What has worked in the past can inform the present and the
future in medicine.

Even when this desirable situation becomes a reality, however, people
will still have the same problem they do today, finding someone who is
compatible with their own personalities, a doctor to whom they can relate
and even trust with the care of their bodies and their medical needs. When
mainstream doctors stop being dismissive of natural approaches and join
alternative practitioners in encouraging their patients to practice prevention by eating well, exercising, and using supplements and herbs to replace
what their food, air, and water are not providing, then these patients will
be able to see their doctors less often and, hopefully, avoid serious illness.

We are, I believe, in both an early, as well as a transitional, stage in
the history of complementary medicine. Compared to those with more conventional views, we are not a large community of physicians, but I know
we represent the future of health and medical care, simply because it
makes sense. Western medical school training gave us our foundation, but
out in the world we discovered there were other approaches to healing
that worked equally well, and some even better. The search was on for
treatments that worked with few, if any, side effects.

A necessary aspect of any transition is that new thinking, new
processes, and new systems exist with the old, which forces both the old
and the new to clarify their beliefs, present them to each other, and struggle with any discrepancies. I understand that the result of this transition
could be a kind of medicine I do not recognize as conventional or complementary. I am equally certain, however, that the principles we espouse will
ultimately outweigh those currently given precedence and will form the
basis of medicine in the twenty-second century. The tools of our craft will

be streamlined. The equipment will be easier to use, more functional. Many of the diseases of today will not exist, replaced by other diseases as yet undeveloped. But the ability of the human body to heal itself will be dramatically enhanced. And the time it takes for that to happen will be miraculously shorter. Most important, the unorthodox concepts and ideas that we as complementary physicians believe in today will be commonplace.

The oxygen therapies I have been discussing in this book are treatments that I know will be even more important at the end of this century. Today, complementary physicians like myself use them as our first line of defense against illness. The work of visionary physicians like Dr. Richard Neubauer was dismissed for most of the twentieth century, but his continuing belief in the efficacy of hyperbaric oxygen therapy is finally being taken seriously. The modality has been in existence for more than 300 years, and enlightened physicians, researchers, and patients who have benefited from treatment with it have kept it from disappearing. In light of the concerted efforts to keep it from becoming a viable treatment in this country, the increasing awareness of its usefulness is somewhat miraculous.

The fact that many doctors are unaware of hyperbaric oxygen therapy's ability to force oxygen into the tissues of the body, directly into the blood plasma (which usually fails to carry oxygen), basically means they are ignorant of an important avenue for healing. Many different diseases, from cancer to chronic fatigue, improve with treatment and *without* side effects. These diseases damage circulation through the capillaries that connect arteries to veins and prevent oxygen from reaching the tissue. HBOT, oxygen under pressure, can override this by infusing the entire body with increased amounts of oxygen. It is a very simple concept, using a natural element rather than a pharmaceutically manufactured substance. The only real expense of the treatment is in the manufacture of the chambers needed.

How long will it take for the medical community and the insurance carriers to understand the advantages of installing a small hyperbaric chamber in every ambulance to treat emergency cases of carbon monoxide poisoning or stroke? It could save so many human lives each year. And the quality of those lives could be vastly improved simply by widening the horizons of medicine's narrow vision. For example, physicians overwhelmingly believe that autism is both untreatable and incurable. But my small study on the treatment of two autistic boys discussed in Chapter 4 should encourage my colleagues to consider the potential for HBOT to make a difference in the lives of autistic children and their families.

In the marketplace of treatment choices, currently dominated by pharmaceutical companies and their advertising agencies, a simple treatment such as HBOT tends to be overlooked because, once bought and paid for, the chambers and the oxygen are basically free. What the patient pays for is the upkeep of the equipment and the professional time of the monitoring physician. That, in the end, will be what insures the future of this particular oxygen therapy, however. It is a relatively inexpensive way to make a difference in the health of patients. Is it a cure in all cases? No, of course not. But it is a treatment that improves most conditions for which it is appropriate, allowing people to return to normal functioning. I predict that, within the next twenty years, the number of HBOT chambers available for use will increase dramatically, bringing down the cost of treatments. Most municipal hospitals already have one installed, but they will need to buy several more when insurance decides to pay for less common uses of the therapy.

Complementary physicians all over the world have accumulated experience and a number of research and clinical studies on hydrogen peroxide therapy and ultraviolet irradiation of blood. The simple methodology and the positive effects of these treatments are gaining fast recognition, particularly in treating the symptoms of people with intractable diseases such as HIV/AIDS and cancer, and contributing greatly to prolonging their health and maintaining a positive quality of life. If ever there were any treatments slated to make a difference in this century, it would be these two oxygen therapies, simple concepts whose use has improved the health of the majority of people treated.

The methodology for applying these treatments is fast, and the equipment is portable and relatively inexpensive. On the other hand, because HBOT requires the use of hyperbaric chambers large enough to accommodate a person, and demands a large enough space in which to install the equipment, it doesn't have the flexibility of H_2O_2 and UVIB treatments, both around for almost a century and, like HBOT, not new. In hydrogen peroxide therapy, H_2O_2 needs to be injected into a vein, and with ultraviolet irradiation of blood, two injections are needed—one to remove a small amount of blood and the other to reinject the blood back into the body once it is exposed to UV light. For some people, that is a problem. Simple, yes, but if you have an aversion to injections, the idea of H_2O_2 or light therapy could be unsettling. Overcoming this natural resistance is a matter of education, which I hope I have accomplished in this book. Once people feel better, they have few problems with the injecting. But I understand that reading about it, or hearing about it, particularly when the substance and method are unfamiliar even to most physicians, and are scarcely mentioned in medical books and journals, can be frightening. My hope is that people who can benefit from these treatments will be able to overcome their fear long enough to experience improvement.

The fact that H_2O_2 and UVIB therapy produce almost no side effects is impressive. As Americans seek simpler and more effective solutions to the health problems of our times, these therapies, alone or working together, can keep patients out of hospitals and enhance their quality of life.

In third world countries, where inexpensive, easily accessible solutions to health problems are greatly needed, treatments such as H_2O_2 and UVIB—portable, easy to understand, easy to apply, and effective—will be invaluable. It is my experience that, the more advanced the society, and the more options it has, the longer it may take for public recognition and governmental support to be forthcoming. So it is logical that our research pool will come from outside the United States. Documentation will be necessary, so follow-up studies are essential for learning more about what kind of treatment program best serves the needs of those with differing conditions and illnesses.

Still considered experimental in the United States, medical ozone looks promising for greater distribution and use in the twenty-first century. Since World War II, the Germans, long-time advocates of ozone use for medical purposes, have been conducting research on it, which continues to this day. Scientists in both Cuba and Russia have taken ozone therapy seriously and have been supported by their governments who advocate universal healthcare. Ozone, inexpensive to produce and an effective therapy in the treatment of many diseases and health conditions, meets the criteria of governments that shy away from private drug manufacturers whose products are far too expensive for countries where socialized medicine prevails. Portable medical ozone generators are available in many parts of the world and are particularly useful in treating people in isolated areas.

I believe that the government-supported research going on today in socialist countries will eventually be the studies that will turn the tide in the United States. As it becomes clearer that, even in the United States, the cost of technology-based healthcare is becoming stratospheric and unaffordable to even the middle class, government support of effective oxygen therapies will start to happen. With that support, the private sector will see an advantage to manufacturing the equipment necessary. And when insurance companies discover that, in the long run, paying for oxygen therapies is more cost-effective than paying for many of the expensive pharmaceutical treatments and surgical procedures currently in use, things will change. I expect that to happen in the twenty-first century.

Although I have concentrated on the remarkable power of bio-oxidative therapies in this book, as a complementary physician, I know that the health of the body/mind is an individual issue, a complicated tangle of the physical, emotional, psychological, and even spiritual aspects of every human being. Diseases can result from any combination of these aspects. The mind's ability to enhance the immune system, and the ability of positive thinking to improve a disease state are no longer wishful thinking. Researchers have proven that negative states of mind, such as anger, fear, and hopelessness, all contribute to ill health, if not disease. I see it every day in my office. The initial visit, sometimes as long as an hour or an hour and a half, is often spent trying to dispel the negativity, to place these new patients, if not in a neutral state, at least in a state where they can hear that change is possible and believe it. It is also why I so often recommend one, or sometimes two, oxygen therapies right away. The infusion of oxygen into their bodies gives them new vitality. They are less pessimistic, less depressed, and more hopeful. And, in such a state, healing can begin.

Today, skepticism is fashionable. I am the last-resort doctor. After the specialists and conventional physicians have implied that there's nothing more to be done, people find me, usually through friends or my radio show. And when they arrive in my office for the first time, they do not, for the most part, believe they will be helped, nor do they believe I can help them. But skeptical people are intelligent people. Why should they believe they can feel better when they have personally experienced failure at the hands of other doctors? So it becomes my challenge, and the challenge of all of us who practice this art called complementary medicine, to prove to them that there is an answer to their problem. Maybe it won't happen overnight, but people who have lived with illness for a long time are very much in tune with their bodies and can detect the smallest difference. So, with each improvement, they can allow themselves to hope they will feel well, really well, one day. People are patient when they feel there is progress in their journey to health.

That is why I say that the most important change in medicine today is attitude. Openness to the possibility that we can be healthy in a way that is compatible to being human is a twenty-first-century concept. And so is the concept that, as individuals, we are in charge of our own bodies and of what happens to them. This change has not happened from the top down. It is people-driven. And it relies on the knowledge that the ideal way to sustain our health is for our bodies to have access to pure air, fresh water, and natural food without pesticides and chemicals. Even if not practiced today, this awareness is accepted as fact and will continue to be by more and more people in the near future. These elements *are* medicine.

Oxygen comes to the rescue, because it is oxygen that sustains all life and will do so as long as there is an Earth. As a complementary physician, I have learned not to take the remarkable potential for healing in the natural world for granted, and I urge you to also keep an open mind about twenty-first-century treatments that may seem unorthodox. Use your common sense, and if it works and you feel better, it is not your imagination working overtime!

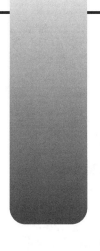

Appendix A

BIO-OXIDATIVE ORGANIZATIONS

International Bio-Oxidative Medicine Association (IBOMF)
P.O. Box 891954
Oklahoma City, Oklahoma 73189-2954
Phone: (405) 634-1310 • Fax: (405) 634-7320

IBOMF was established in 1987 for the purposes of research and education in the field of oxidative medicine. The referral list below is organized by state. IBOMF does not provide information or recommendations about specific medical problems or questions, nor does it recommend any product or equipment. However, its membership is knowledgeable about the treatments discussed in this book, including hydrogen peroxide therapy, hyperbaric oxygen therapy, ozone therapy, and ultraviolet irradiation of blood. Not all members use all of these oxygen therapies in their practice, so if you are interested in a specific therapy, it would be wise to query the practitioner before making an appointment.

This following list is from the IBOMF membership, as presented on their website. If you are interested in oxygen therapy, this is a good place to begin your research. (Phone numbers and addresses subject to change.)

The asterisk denotes the practitioners who have completed workshop training and written exams, and have been awarded Diplomate Status.

Alaska

Robert Rowen, M.D.*
615 East 82nd St., Suite #300
Anchorage, Alaska 99518
Phone: (907) 344-7775
Fax: (907) 622-3114

Arkansas

Melissa Taliaferro, M.D.*
P.O. Box 400
Leslie, Arkansas 72645
Phone: (501) 447-2599
Fax: (501) 447-2917

Arizona

Terry Friedman, M.D.
10565 N. Tatum Blvd., Suite B-115
Paradise Valley, Arizona 85254
Phone: (602) 381-0800

Thomas J. Grade, M.D.
6644 East Baywood Ave.
Mesa, Arizona 85206
Phone: (602) 981-4474
Fax: (602) 981-4312

California

John Beneck, M.D.
22107 Old Paint Way
Canyon Lake, California 92587
Phone: (909) 244-3686
Fax: (909) 244-0109

Nola Higa, M.D.
221 Town Center West, #101
Santa Maria, California 93454
Phone: (805) 347-0067
Fax: (805) 909-3032

Robert M. Martin, M.D.
2015 East Florence Ave.
Los Angeles, California 90001
Phone: (213) 277-9096
Fax: (213) 277-9098

Martin Mulders, M.D.*
3301 Alta Arden, #3
Sacramento, California 95825
Phone: (916) 489-4400
Fax: (916) 489-1710

Francis V. Pau, M.D.
1465 Loma Sola Court
Upland, California 91786
Phone: (909) 987-4262
Fax: (909) 987-9542

David A. Steenblock, D.O.
26381 Crown Valley Pkwy.,
  Suite 130
Mission Viejo, California 92691
Phone: (714) 367-8870
Fax: (714) 770-9775

Thomas R. Yarema, M.D.
1218 Monroe Ave.
San Diego, California 92116
Phone: (619) 299-8607
Fax: (619) 299-8671

Colorado

Terry Grossman, M.D.
255 Union St., #400
Lakewood, Colorado 80228

Thomas R. Lawrence, D.C.
2222 East 18th Ave.
Denver, Colorado 80206
Phone: (303) 333-3733
Fax: (303) 333-1352

Florida

Naima Abdel-Ghany, M.D.
340 West 23rd St., Suite E
Panama City, Florida 32405
Phone: (904) 763-7689

Gary L. Pynkel, D.O., M.D.*
3840 Colonial Blvd, Suite #1
Fort Myers, Florida 33912
Phone: (941) 278-3377

Martin Dayton, D.O.*
18600 Collins Avenue
North Miami Beach, Florida 33160
Phone: (305) 931-8484

William Campbell Douglass
III, M.D.
101 Timberlachen, Suite 101
Lake Mary, Florida 32746
Phone: (407) 324-0888
Fax: (407) 324-8222

Nelson Kraucek, M.D.
8923 NE 134th Ave., Suite A
Lady Lake, Florida 32159
Phone: (352) 750-4333
Fax: (352) 750-2023

Eteri Melnikov, M.D.
116 Manatee Ave. E.
Braden River, Florida 34208
Phone: (813) 748-7943

Carlos A. Unzueta, M.D.
1204 Carlton Ave.
Lake Wales, Florida 33853
Phone: (941) 676-7569
Fax: (941) 676-3896

William N. Watson, M.D.
5536 Stewart St., NE
Milton, Florida 32570
Phone: (904) 623-3836
Fax: (904) 623-2201

Georgia

Martin L. Bremer, D.O.
P.O. Box 131
Cornelia, Georgia 30531
Phone: (770) 538-0910
Fax: (770) 538-0910

Milton Fried, M.D.
4426 Tilly Mill Rd.
Atlanta, Georgia 30360
Phone: (770) 451-4857
Fax: (770) 451-8492

Oliver E. Gunter, M.D.
P.O. Box 347
Camilla, Georgia 31730
Phone: (912) 336-7343
Fax: (912) 336-7400

Hawaii

Wendell Foo, M.D.
2357 S. Beratania St., A-349
Honolulu, Hawaii 96826
Phone: (808) 373-4007

Idaho

Patrick H. Ranch, D.C.,
M.D., N.M.D.
810 North Henry, #230
Post Falls, Idaho, 83854
Phone: (208) 777-8297

Illinois

Robert Filice, M.D.
1280 Iroquois Dr., #200
Naperville, Illinois 60563
Phone: (708) 386-0078
Fax: (708) 848-7789

Thomas L. Hesselink, M.D.
888 S. Edgelawn Dr., Suite #1743
Aurora, Illinois 60506
Phone: (708) 844-0011
Fax: (708) 844-0500

William J. Mauer, D.O.*
3401 N. Kennicot Ave., Suite #800
Arlington Heights, Illinois 60005
Phone: (708) 255-8988
Fax: (708) 255-7700

Kansas

Jerry E. Block, M.D., F.A.C.P.
1501 West 4th St.
Coffeyville, Kansas 67337
Phone: (316) 251-2400
Fax: (316) 251-1619

Kentucky

Ralph G. Ellis, M.D.
112 Stone House Trail
Bardstown, Kentucky 40004
Phone/Fax: (502) 349-6313

Massachusetts

Denise D. Cantin, D.O.
415 Boston Tpke., Route #9
Shrewsbury, Massachusetts
  01545
Phone: (508) 842-8118
Fax: (508) 842-2148

Michael Janson, M.D.
18 Bond Street
Cambridge, Massachusetts
  02138
Phone: (617) 547-0295

Maine

Arthur B. Weisser, D.O.
184 Silver St.
Waterville, Maine 04901
Phone: (207) 873-7721
Fax: (207) 873-7724

Michigan

Vahagn Agbabian, D.O.*
28 Saginaw St., Suite #1105
Pontiac, Michigan 48058
Phone: (810) 334-2424
Fax: (810) 258-0488

Missouri

Ralph Cooper, D.O.
1608 East 20th St.
Joplin, Missouri 64804
Phone: (417) 624-4323

Harvey Walker, Jr., M.D. Ph.D.
138 North Meramac Ave.
St. Louis, Missouri 63105
Phone: (314) 721-7227
Fax: (314) 721-7247

Nebraska

Otis Miller, M.D.
1001 South 14th St.
Ord, Nebraska 68862
Phone: (308) 728-3251

Nevada

Robert D. Milne, M.D.
2110 Pinto Lane
Las Vegas, Nevada 89106
Phone: (702) 385-1393
Fax: (702) 385-4170

North Carolina

John C. Pittman, M.D.*
4505 Fair Meadow Lane, #111
Raleigh, North Carolina 27622
Phone: (919) 571-4391
Fax: (919) 571-8968

New Jersey

Stuart Weg, M.D.*
1250 East Ridgewood Ave.
Ridgewood, New Jersey 07450
Phone: (201) 447-5558
Fax: (201) 447-9011

New York

Richard Ash, M.D.
800 5th Ave.
New York, New York 10021
Phone: (212) 628-3113
Fax: (212) 249-3805

Kenneth A. Bock, M.D.*
108 Montgomery St.
Rhinebeck, New York 12472
Phone: (914) 876-7082
Fax: (914) 876-4615

Mitchell Kurk, M.D.*
310 Broadway
Lawrence, New York 11555
Phone: (516) 239-5540
Fax: (516) 371-2919

Joyce H. Marshall, N.D.
23 Madison St.
Hamilton, New York 13346
Phone: (315) 824-3007

Bruce D. Oran, D.O.
Two Executive Blvd., Suite #202
Suffern, New York 10901
Phone: (914) 368-4700
Fax: (914) 368-4727

Robert W. Snider, M.D.
284 Andrews St.
Massena, New York 13662
Phone: (315) 764-0997
Fax: (315) 769-6713

Michael J. Teplitsky, M.D.
415 Oceanview Ave.
Brooklyn, New York 11235
Phone: (718) 769-0997
Fax: (718) 646-2352

Richard J. Ucci, M.D.*
521 Main St.
Oneonta, New York 13820
Phone: (607) 431-9641

Pavel I. Yutsis, M.D.
The CAM Institute for Integrative
   Therapies
264 First St.
Brooklyn, New York 11215
Phone: (718) 768-4505
Fax: (718) 768-2496

Ohio

John Baron, D.O.
4807 Rockside Rd., Suite #100
Cleveland, Ohio 43203
Phone: (216) 642-0082
Fax: (216) 642-1415

Bruce Massau, D.O., E.M.B.A.
1470-B Hawthorne Ave.
Columbus, Ohio 43203
Phone: (614) 252-1500
Fax: (614) 252-1685

James C. Roberts, M.D.
4607 Sylvania Ave., Suite #200
Toledo, Ohio 43623
Phone: (419) 882-9620
Fax: (419) 882-9628

Sherri Tenpenny, D.O.
13550 Falling Waters Rd.
Strongsville, Ohio 44136
Phone: (216) 572-1136
Fax: (216) 572-2195

Oklahoma

Leon Anderson, D.O.*
121 South Second St.
Jenks, Oklahoma 74037
Phone: (918) 299-5038
Fax: (918) 299-5030

Charles Hathaway, D.C.
1607 South Muskogee Ave.
Tahlequah, Oklahoma 74464
Phone: (918) 456-8090
Fax: (918) 456-6060

James W. Hogin, D.O.
937 S.W. 89th St., Suite #C
Oklahoma City, Oklahoma
   73139
Phone: (405) 631-0524
Fax: (405) 631-9465

Gordon P. Laird, D.O.
304 Boulder St.
Pawnee, Oklahoma 74058
Phone: (918) 762-3601
Fax: (918) 762-2544

Maged H. Maged, M.D.*
5419 S. Western Ave.
Oklahoma City, Oklahoma
   73109
Phone: (405) 634-7855
Fax: (405) 634-7320

Richard Santelli, D.C.*
9216 N.W. 104th St.
Oklahoma City, Oklahoma
   73109
Phone: (405) 789-5114

Charles Taylor, M.D.
3715 N. Classen Blvd.
Oklahoma City, Oklahoma
   73118
Phone: (405) 525-7751
Fax: (405) 747-2717

Michael Taylor, D.C.
3808 E. 51st St.
Tulsa, Oklahoma 74119
Phone: (918) 749-4657
Fax: (918) 749-6263

Robert L. White, Ph.D., N.D.
5419 S. Western Ave.
Oklahoma City, Oklahoma
   73109
Phone: (405) 634-7855
Fax: (405) 634-7320

Oregon

Robert Jamison, M.D.
628 Pacific Terrace
Klamath Falls, Oregon 97601

J. Stephen Schaub, M.D.
9310 S.E. Stark St.
Portland, Oregon 97216
Phone: (503) 256-9666

Pennsylvania

Harold Buttram, M.D.*
5724 Clymer Rd.
Quakertown, Pennsylvania
   18951
Phone: (215) 536-1890
Fax: (215) 529-9034

Arthur Koch, D.O.*
57 West Juniper St.
Hazelton, Pennsylvania 18201
Phone: (717) 455-4747
Fax: (717) 455-6312

John M. Sullivan, M.D.
1001 South Market St., Suite #B
Mechanicsburg, Pennsylvania
   17055
Phone: (717) 697-5050

Texas

Antonio Acevedo, M.D.
P.O. Box 707
Bedford, Texas 76021
Phone: (817) 595-2580
Fax: (817) 589-2913

Robert M. Battle, M.D.
9910 Long Point Rd.
Houston, Texas 77055
Phone: (713) 932-0552
Fax: (713) 932-0551

Ronald W. Bowen, D.O.
7121 S. Padre Island Dr., Suite #104
Corpus Christi, Texas 78412
Phone: (512) 985-1115
Fax: (512) 985-1467

Patricia Braun, M.D.
1212 Coit Rd., Suite #110
Piano, Texas TP2 75075
Phone: (214) 612-0399
Fax: (214) 985-1207

Elisabeth Ann Cole, M.D.*
1002 Brockman Rd.
Sweeney, Texas 77480
Phone: (409) 548-8610
Fax: (409) 549-8614

Ronald M. Davis, M.D.
5002 Toddville Rd.
Seabrook, Texas 77586
Phone: (713) 474-3495

John Galewaler, D.O.
P.O. Box 488
Celina, Texas 75009
Phone: (214) 382-2345

Charles M. Hawes, D.O.*
6451 Brentwood Stair Rd., Suite #115
Fort Worth, Texas 76112
Phone: (817) 446-8416
Fax: (817) 446-8413

T. Roger Humphrey, M.D.
2400 Rushing St.
Wichita Falls, Texas 76308
Phone: (817) 766-4329
Fax: (817) 767-3227

George Lofgren, N.D.
1220 Town East Blvd., #250B
Mesquite, Texas 75150
Phone: (214) 636-2696
Fax: (214) 635-9238

James J. Mahoney, D.O.
6451 Brentwood Stair Rd.,
   Suite #115
Fort Worth, Texas 76112
Phone: (817) 446-8416
Fax: (817) 446-8413

Ron Manzanero, M.D.
3845 F.M. 2222, #23
Austin, Texas 78731
Phone: (512) 258-1647
Fax: (512) 453-3450

Frank J. Morales, Jr. M.D.*
2805 Hackberry Rd.
Brownsville, Texas 78521
Phone: (210) 504-2330
Fax: (210) 548-1227

Carlos Nossa, M.D.
4010 Fairmont Pkwy., #274
Pasadena, Texas 77504
Phone: (713) 334-1456

Benjamin Thurman, M.D.
102 North Magdalen St., #290
San Angelo, Texas 76903
Phone: (915) 653-3562
Fax: (915) 944-1162

Barbara Weeden, C.C.N.
800 Secretary Dr.
Arlington, Texas 76015
Phone: (817) 265-5261
Fax: (817) 274-9971

Utah

Dennis Harper, D.O.*
5263 S. 300 W, #203
Murray, Utah 84107
Phone: (801) 288-8881
Fax: (801) 262-4860

Washington

Patrick H. Ranch, M.D., D.C.
9629 North Indian Trail Rd.
Spokane, Washington 99208
Phone: (208) 777-8297
Fax: (208) 466-6043

There are a number of international members as well, located mostly in Canada, also in the United Kingdom, the Phillipines, Malaysia, and Africa. Their addresses, phone numbers, and fax numbers can be accessed on the Internet.

CHOOSING A THERAPIST

One of the most difficult aspects of getting oxygen therapy is choosing a practitioner. It is as difficult as selecting a conventional medical doctor. Personal recommendations are clearly the best source, but in alternative medicine, such recommendations are not easily available. I suggest querying the professional, personally if possible and, if not, asking for written information on the physician or practitioner's background regarding the number of years in practice, the type of equipment available, and the number of patients he/she has treated. Then use your intuitive sense of whether the practitioner is forthcoming, knowledgeable, and someone with whom you would like to work. It has been my experience in dealing with new physicians that the first contact is with the staff of the office. Doctors who hire considerate, intelligent, helpful staff usually share those qualities themselves. If you feel uncomfortable or uneasy with a medical practitioner—conventional or complementary—my advice is to look elsewhere.

HYPERBARIC OXYGEN THERAPY

For information on hyperbaric oxygen therapy, contact the following two organizations:

**The American College of
  Hyperbaric Medicine**
(through The Ocean Hyperbaric Center)
4001 Ocean Dr.
Lauderdale-by-the-Sea,
  Florida 33308
Phone: (954) 771-4000
Fax: (954) 776-0670

**Undersea Hyperbaric Medical
  Society, Inc.**
10531 Metropolitan Ave.
Kensington, Maryland 20895-2627
Phone: (301) 942-2980
Fax: (301) 942-7804
E-mail: uhmn@radix.net
Website: http://www.umhs.org

HYDROGEN PEROXIDE THERAPY

Any of the practitioners whose names appear in the above listing of medical professionals can answer your questions on hydrogen peroxide therapy. It is a common treatment known by all complementary physicians and used by most of them. Intravenous hydrogen peroxide is a basic method of increasing oxygen to the cells as a therapeutic treatment. Its most useful quality is that H_2O_2 can be used with almost any therapy to treat most diseases.

ULTRAVIOLET IRRADIATION OF BLOOD

For information specifically on photoluminescence, or UVIB therapy, contact the following organization for centers in your area.

Foundation for Blood Irradiation
1315 Apple Ave.
Silver Spring, Maryland 20910
Phone: (301) 587-8688
Fax: (301) 587-8686
E-mail: uv@uvbl.com
Website: http//users.erols.com/mrfinc/ubi10b.html

The source for this information comes from the Wellness Directory of Minnesota, phone: (763) 689-9355.

OZONE THERAPY

For specific information on centers performing the therapy, or for further education on the subject, contact the following organization.

The International Ozone Association, Inc.
Pan American Group
31 Strawberry Hill Ave.
Stamford, Connecticut 06902
Phone: (203) 348-3542
Fax: (203) 967-4845
Website: www.int-ozone-assoc.org/

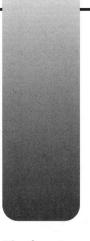

Appendix B

THERAPEUTIC USES FOR VARIOUS OXYGEN THERAPIES

The four oxygen therapies I have discussed in this book are, as you now know, in the process of continuing exploration. They are used independently or in combination for maximum impact. Although the conditions they treat have been listed throughout the book, I felt it would be useful for the reader to see the numbers of conditions and diseases that are candidates for these various therapies listed together. Your complementary physician can tell you which of these therapies, or what combination of therapies, will best serve you and help rebalance your body and make improvements to your general health. You can also use this book as a means of introducing the subject to your physician.

HYPERBARIC OXYGEN THERAPY (HBOT)

Hyperbaric oxygen therapy has been used to treat the following conditions.[1] As with the other oxygen therapies, the treatment has varying degrees of success depending on the patient's health. However, most of these conditions have benefited from hyperbaric oxygen, alone or in combination with other oxygen therapies. Dr. Neubauer and Dr. Walker point out that HBOT may be especially beneficial when other measures have failed.

Emergency Indications

Air embolism
Blast injury
Burns
Carbon monoxide
  poisoning
Cerebral edema
Closed head injuries

Crisis of sickle cell
  anemia
Decompression
  sickness
Gas gangrene
Hydrogen sulfide
  poisoning

Near-drowning
Near-electrocution
Near-hanging
Peyote poisoning
Severed limbs
Smoke inhalation
Ileus

Neurologic Indications

Acute and chronic stroke
Air embolism
Cerebral edema
Cranial nerve syndromes
Early organic brain syndrome
Multiple sclerosis
Peripheral neuropathy
Spinal cord contusion
Vegetative coma

Orthopedic Indications

Acute and chronic osteomyelitis
Acute necrotizing fasciitis
Aseptic necrosis
Bone grafting
Clostridial myonecrosis
Compartment syndrome
Crush injuries
Delayed wound healing
Edema under cast
Fracture nonunion
Severed limbs and digits
Soft tissue swelling
Stump infections
Tendon and ligament injuries,
   postsurgical repair

Miscellaneous Indications

Buerger's disease
Cerebral palsy
Chronic fatigue
Cirrhosis
Crohn's disease
Diabetic retinopathy
Frostbite
Gangrene (wet and dry)
Lepromatous leprosy
Migraine
Myocardial infarction
Peptic ulcer
Peripheral vascular ulcer
Pneumatosis cystoides intestinalis
Post-cardiotomy low output
   failure
Post polio syndrome
Pseudomembranous colitis
Radiation cystitis and enteritis
Refractory mycoses
Retinal artery occlusion
Retinal vein thrombosis
Rheumatoid arthritis, (acute)
   scleroderma
Sickle cell crisis and hematuria

Intravenous Hydrogen Peroxide

Intravenous hydrogen peroxide has been applied to the following conditions with varying degrees of success, depending on the health variables of individual patients.

Acute and chronic viral infections
Arrhythmias
Asthma

Cerebral vascular disease
Coronary spasm (angina)
Cardioconversion

Chronic fatigue syndrome (chronic recurrent Epstein-Barr infection)

Chronic obstructive pulmonary disease

Chronic pain syndromes (multiple causes)

Chronic unresponsive bacterial infection

Cluster headaches

Diabetes type II

Emphysema

Environmental allergy reactions (universal)

Herpes simplex

Herpes zoster

HIV infections

Influenza

Metastatic carcinoma

Migraine headaches

Multiple sclerosis

Parkinsonism

Peripheral vascular disease

Rheumatoid arthritis

Systemic chronic candidiasis

Temporal arteritis

Vascular headaches

Ozone Therapy

Ozone therapy, too, has been used to treat a wide range of conditions.[2] As with the other oxygen therapies, it has been used alone or in combination with other oxygen therapies, with varying degrees of success. Ozone therapy continues to be widely researched around the world, and clinically, the results are very favorable. Indications for use are listed as follows.

Superinfected and Badly Healing Wounds, Inflammatory Processes

Abscess

Anal Fissure

Apthae

Arthritis conditions

Burns plus burn sequels

Candidiasis

Cystitis (molds, discharge)

Decubitus

Dental applications

Discharge

Epidermophytic conditions

Fistulae

Fluor genitalis

Furunculosis

Gangrene

Leg ulcers

Molds

Polyarthritis

Spondylitis

Stomatitiis

Thrush

Ulcus cruris

Circulatory Disorders-Conditions of Older People

Allergies
Arterial Circulatory disorders
Arteriosclerosis
Circulatory disorders
Circulatory disorders (arterials)
Gangrene
Geriatric applications
Hepatitis

Herpes genitalis
Herpes labialis
Herpes zoster
Oncology, additive
Parkinson's disease
Raynaud's disease
Viral diseases

Photoluminescence—Ultraviolet Irradiation of Blood (UVIB)

Photoluminescence, or ultraviolet irradiation of blood, also used alone or in combination with other oxygen therapies, differs from them because with UVIB a portion of a person's blood is removed, exposed to ultraviolet light, and then reinjected into the body, stimulating the immune system. This exciting treatment continues to be researched and has been used in the treatment of the conditions listed below.

Asthma
Autoimmune diseases (rheumatoid
  arthritis, lupus)
Bacterial endocarditis
Cancer (experimentally)
Diphtheria
Emphysema
Food poisoning
Gangrene
HIV/AIDS
Immune deficiency
Inflammatory processes (bursitis,
  fibrositis, iritis, pancreatitis)
Mumps

Non-healing wounds and wound
  infections
Osteomyelitis
Peripheral vascular disease (and
  other vascular conditions)
Peritonitis
Pneumonia
Polio
Septicemia
Thrombophlebitis
Veterinary medicine
Viral infections (hepatitis,
  respiratory)

Oxygen therapies are useful for most medical problems because, as I've pointed out, oxygen's healing potential can generally be applied to almost any condition. However, because they are not yet familiar to many physicians, they are most often used when more conventional treatments fail to produce positive effects.

References

Books

* Denotes recommended reading.

Ali, Majid. *Oxygen and Aging.* New York, NY: Aging Healthfully, Inc., 2000.

Altman, Nathaniel. *Oxygen Healing Therapies.* Foreword by Charles H. Farr. Rochester, VT: Healing Arts Press, 1995.*

Burton Goldberg Group. *Alternative Medicine.* Puyallup, WA: Future Medicine Publishing, Inc., 1993.

Douglass, William Campbell. *Hydrogen Peroxide: Medical Miracle.* Atlanta, GA: Second Opinion Publishing, 1990.*

Douglass, William Campbell. *Into the Light.* Atlanta, GA: Second Opinion Publishing, 1993.*

Ito, Dee. *Without Estrogen: Natural Remedies for Menopause and Beyond.* New York, NY: Crown Publishing, 1994.

Jain, K. K. *Textbook of Hyperbaric Medicine.* "Hyperbaric Oxygen Therapy in Miscellaneous Neurological Disorders," Chapter 19. Springer Publishers, 1995.

McCabe, Ed. *O2xygen Therapies.* 99-RD1, Morrisville, NY 13408: Energy Publications, 1988.*

Neubauer, Richard, Walker, Morton. *Hyperbaric Oxygen Therapy.* Garden City Park, NY: Avery Publishing Group, 1998.*

Oriani, G., Moroni, A., Wattel, S. *Handbook of Hyperbaric Medicine.* New York, NY: Springer Publishing, 1995.

Petrovsky, B.V., Efuni, Sergey. *Basics of Hyperbaric Oxygenation*. Moscow, Russia: Moscow Medicine, 1976.

Reillo, Michelle. *Aids Under Pressure*. Seattle, Washington, Toronto, Canada, Gottingen, Germany, Bern, Switzerland: Hogrefe & Huber Publishers, 1960.*

Viebahn, Renate. *The Use of Ozone in Medicine*. 2nd English Edition, Transl. Andrew Lee. Heidelberg, Germany: Karl F. Haug Publ., 1994.*

Yutsis, Pavel, Toth, Lynda. *Why Can't I Remember?*: Garden City Park, NY: Avery Publishing Group, 1999.

Yutsis, Pavel, Walker, Morton. *The Downhill Syndrome*. Garden City Park, NY: Avery Publishing Group, 1997.

Periodicals

Catalano, Peter. "Breaking Comas." *Natural Science*, October, 1995, 148–155.

International Council for Health Freedom. "Hyperbaric oxygenation coming into its own as safe, effective treatment for vast array of ills." *Newsletter*, June 30, 1999:40–42.

Kent, Heather. "Customers lining up for high cost hyperbaric therapy." *JAMC Journal of the Canadian Medical Association*, April 6, 1999: 1043–1045.

LeBeau, Conrad. *Hydrogen Peroxide*. Pamphlet. *Vita Health Products*. West Allis, WI, 1998.

Neubauer, Richard, Walker, Morton. "Hyperbaric Oxygen Therapy." *The Townsend Letter for Doctors and Patients*. December 31, 1998: 66–70.

Neubauer, Richard A., Yutsis, Pavel. "New Frontiers: Anti-Aging Properties of Hyperbaric Oxygen Therapy." *The Townsend Letter for Doctors and Patients*. July, 1999:68–69.

Walker, Morton. "Medical Journalist Report on Innovative Biologics: Effective Wound Healing with HBOT." *Townsend Letter for Doctors and Patients*. July 31, 1998:66–70.

Yutsis, Pavel. "Conquering the Challenge." *Fibromyalgia Coalition International Newsletter*. July/August/September, 2000:1–2.

Organizations

The Edelson Center for Environmental and Preventive Medicine
Edelson, Stephen B., M.D.
Atlanta, Georgia 30342
Phone: (401) 841-0088
Website: www.edelsoncenter@edelsoncenter.com.

The Foundation for Light Therapy
Articles: "Historical Overview," "Hydrogen Peroxide-Ozone,"
"Oxidative Medicine," "Ultraviolet Light Therapy Summary."
Boca Raton, Florida 33433
Phone: (561) 274-7078
Website: www.FFLT.org.

Keep Hope Alive
P.O. Box 270041
West Allis, WI, 53227
Website: www.keephope.net
Keep Hope Alive is an organization to contact for the most recent information on useful combinations of approaches, including the bio-oxidative therapies.

All of the above are important resources for myself as an author and as the producer and host of *From Allergies to Aging,* a weekly radio on WEVD in Manhattan, with a signal that spans the East Coast.

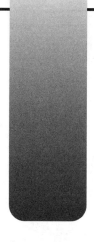

Notes

Introduction

1. Altman, Nathaniel. *Oxygen Healing Therapies*. Rochester, Vermont: Healing Arts Press, 1998. page103.

Chapter 1

1. Douglass, William Campbell. *Into the Light*. Atlanta, GA: Second Opinion Publishing, 1993.

2. *Wholistic Cancer Therapy and Oxygen–Peroxides–Ozone*. Tulsa, OK: Rockland Corporation, 1992, page 6.

Chapter 2

1. Neubauer, Richard A., Walker, Morton. *Hyperbaric Oxygen Therapy*, Garden City Park, NY: Avery Publishing Group, 1998, page 6.

Chapter 4

1. Neubauer, Richard A., Walker, Morton. *Hyperbaric Oxygen Therapy*, Garden City Park, NY: Avery Publishing Group, 1998, page 48.

2. Reillo, Michelle. *Aids Under Pressure*. Case 1. Seattle, Washington, Toronto, Canada, Gottingen, Germany, Bern, Switzerland: Hogrefe & Huber Publishers, 1960, page 47.

3. Neubauer, Richard A., Walker, Morton. *Hyperbaric Oxygen Therapy*, Garden City Park, NY: Avery Publishing Group, 1998, page 70.

4. Neubauer, Richard, Pevsner, Henry, and Gottleib, Sheldon F. Report presented to the International Joint Meeting on Hyperbaric and Underwater Medicine, Milan, Italy, September 8, 1996.

5. Study: "Hyperbaric Treatment in Cerebrovascular Disorders" Dept. of Neurology, Russian Medical University, Moscow, Russia, 1997.

6. James, Philip. "Hyperbaric Oxygen Therapy for Cerebral Palsy Children." Wolfson Hyperbaric Medicine Unit, The University of Dundee, Ninewells Medical School, Dundee, Scotland, 1995.

7. Plank, Trish. "Hyperbaric Oxygen Therapy: Adjunctive Role in the Treatment of Autism." Hyperbaric Centers of Reno, NV and Santa Monica, CA.

Chapter 5

1. Altman, Nathaniel. *Oxygen Healing Therapies.* Foreword by Charles H. Farr. Rochester, VT: Healing Arts Press, 1995, page 59.

2. To read more about the Yutsis FAVER diet, see *The Downhill Syndrome* by Pavel Yutsis, and Morton Walker. Garden City Park, NY: Avery Publishing Group, 1997, pages 84–85.

Chapter 6

1. Altman, Nathaniel. *Oxygen Healing Therapies.* Foreword by Charles H. Farr. Rochester, VT: Healing Arts Press, 1995, page 54.

Chapter 7

1. Viebahn, Renate. *The Use of Ozone in Medicine.* Second American Edition, transl. Andrew Lee. Heidelberg, Germany: Karl F. Haug Publishers, 1994, page 14.

Chapter 8

1. The Foundation for Light Therapy is a non-profit group formed for scientific, educational, charitable, and humanitarian purposes, which promotes the wider use of light energy and oxygen therapies. Boca Raton, Florida. Phone: (561) 274-7078. Their Internet address is wwwFFLT.org.

2. On September 11, 1928, Emmett Knott received patent #1, 683, 877 for "Means for Treating Bloodstream Infections," a UV apparatus that he built. On January 19, 1943, he received a second patent, #2,308,516, for changes to the original equipment. The machine received FDA grandfather status as a device sold and distributed in interstate commerce prior to 1976.

3. Douglass, William Campbell. *Into the Light.* Atlanta, GA: Second Opinion Publishing, 1993, page 23.

4. Douglass, William Campbell. *Into the Light.* Atlanta, GA: Second Opinion Publishing, 1993, page 35.

Chapter 9

1. Douglass, William Campbell. *Into the Light.* Atlanta, GA: Second Opinion Publishing, 1993, page 250.

2. Douglass, William Campbell. *Into the Light.* Atlanta, GA: Second Opinion Publishing, 1993, page 100.

Chapter 10

1. Reillo, Michelle. *Aids Under Pressure.* Seattle, Washington, Toronto, Canada, Gottingen, Germany, Bern, Switzerland: Hogrefe & Huber Publishing, 1960, page 1.

Conclusion

1. Harvard University seminar on Complementary and Integrative Medicine. Under Epidemiology, A. "Prevalence, Costs, and Patterns of Use of CAM Therapies in the United States." March 24–26, 2002, page 4.

Appendix B

1. This list is excerpted from *Hyperbaric Oxygen Therapy* by Richard Neubauer, M.D., and Morton Walker, Garden City Park, NY: Avery Publishing Group, 1998.

2. List synthesized from *The Use of Ozone In Medicine* by Renate Viebahn. English Edition Translated from the German by Andrew Lee. Karl F. Haug Publishers, Heidelberg, Germany, 1987.

Index

About the Author

Pavel Yutsis is a complementary physician, board certified in oxidative medicine, naturopathic medicine, and chelation therapy. A member of the American College for the Advancement in Medicine, the American Academy of Preventive Medicine, and the American Academy of Environmental Medicine, he is the Medical Director of the CAM Institute for Integrative Therapies in Brooklyn, New York. Dr. Yutsis hosts his own radio show, *From Allergies To Aging,* which is widely listened to in the Northeast, and he has authored numerous articles for such publications as the *Journal of Longevity Research, Explore Magazine,* and *To Your Health.* He is the co-author of *The Downhill Syndrome* and *Why Can't I Remember?* Dr. Yutsis lives in the New York City area with his wife and two children.